Cool Connections with Cognitive Behavioural Therapy for Groups

in the same series

Cool Connections CBT Workbook
Build Your Self-Esteem, Resilience and Well-Being for Ages 9–14
Laurie Seiler
Illustrated by Adam Alan Freeman
ISBN 978 1 78775 254 2
eISBN 978 1 78775 255 9

of related interest

Creative Coping Skills for Teens and Tweens
Activities for Self Care and Emotional Support including Art, Yoga, and Mindfulness
Bonnie Thomas
ISBN 978 1 78592 814 7
eISBN 978 1 78450 888 3

The Mental Health and Wellbeing Workout for Teens
Skills and Exercises from ACT and CBT for Healthy Thinking
Paula Nagel
Illustrated by Gary Bainbridge
ISBN 978 1 78592 394 4
eISBN 978 1 78450 753 4

CBT Doodling for Kids
50 Illustrated Handouts to Help Build Confidence and
Emotional Resilience in Children Aged 6–11
Tanja Sharpe
ISBN 978 1 78592 537 5
eISBN 978 1 78775 017 3

Cool Connections with Cognitive Behavioural Therapy for Groups

2nd edition

Encouraging Self-Esteem, Resilience and Well-Being in Children and Young People Using CBT Approaches

LAURIE SEILER

Illustrated by Adam Alan Freeman

Jessica Kingsley Publishers
London and Philadelphia

First published in Great Britain in 2021 by Jessica Kingsley Publishers
An Hachette Company

1

Copyright © Laurie Seiler 2021
Illustrations copyright © Adam Alan Freeman 2021

A CIP catalogue record for this title is available from the
British Library and the Library of Congress

ISBN 978 1 78775 247 4
eISBN 978 1 78775 248 1

Printed and bound in Great Britain by TJ International Ltd.

Jessica Kingsley Publishers' policy is to use papers that are natural, renewable and recyclable products and made from wood grown in sustainable forests. The logging and manufacturing processes are expected to conform to the environmental regulations of the country of origin.

Jessica Kingsley Publishers
73 Collier Street
London N1 9BE, UK

www.jkp.com

MIX
Paper from
responsible sources
FSC® C013056
FSC
www.fsc.org

Contents

Preface

I would like to share a little information about myself, the Cool Connections Programme and its development. Having worked for a number of years within the caring professions, I qualified as a mental health nurse at Brunel University in 1997. Since then I have acquired a BSc (Hons) in specialist practice, a BA (Hons) in child and adolescent mental health studies, and a postgraduate diploma in cognitive behavioural therapy (CBT). I am also a fully accredited cognitive behavioural psychotherapist and registered with the British Association for Behavioural and Cognitive Psychotherapies (BABCP).

The Cool Connections Programme outlined in this book is an early intervention group programme aimed at children aged 9–14. The programme is based on a cognitive behavioural approach and focuses on the prevention of anxiety and depression in children and young people. Included in this book is a facilitators' guide, which describes how to run the programme. Referral forms and home activity exercises are also included. The 13 sessions are all illustrated and involve games, theory and numerous fun exercises.

My interest in creating a group programme for young people first developed following my work with children and families in Suffolk. Although there are several books with both interesting and creative ways of working with children, most focus either on older children or on young people with serious mental health difficulties, rather than on early intervention. Many of the exercises in the programme were developed through trial and error and following evaluation by the many children who have taken part.

The first edition of the programme was published in 2008. Since then, there has been a lot of interest in the programme, and the book has been published in different languages around the world. There have also been advances in CBT treatment since 2008, and I have trained in both neuro-linguistic programming (NLP) and eye movement desensitisation reprogramming (EMDR), learning transferable skills which can be used with young people within a cognitive behavioural formulation or framework. This has informed the second edition of the programme, bringing it up to date with the latest research and making it more comprehensive than ever before.

This new second edition includes useful resources aimed at helping children cope with uncomfortable emotions and feelings. It also includes a chapter on mindfulness, and various skills adapted from behavioural activation, acceptance and commitment therapy (ACT) and compassion-based therapies.

Acknowledgements

My thanks go to Dr Nicola Ridgeway and Sue Darker-Smith who have supervised my practice over the past few years and with whom I have shared many ideas for the programme. Also to John Plester, who provided me with training in NLP. My good friend Ashley Barber has helped me with some of the IT ideas and computer technology. Thanks also to all members of the On Track team in Suffolk who supported me in putting the first edition of this programme together, along with the many helpful comments made by the children who have taken part over the years. Teachers Amy Arnold and Rachel Bacon have also been very helpful with updating the second edition with regard to the curriculum and useful ways of implementing early intervention strategies in primary school settings.

Group Facilitators' Guide to the Cool Connections Programme

Cool Connections is a 13-session early intervention programme aimed at children aged 9–14. The programme is based on a cognitive behavioural approach which aims to encourage self-esteem, social skills and well-being, and prevent anxiety and depression in children and adolescents.

THE GROUP FACILITATORS

The programme is written for those qualified to work with children, such as healthcare professionals, psychologists, teachers, social workers and youth counsellors. Unqualified staff can also facilitate the programme but they should spend time discussing and planning the group at least once every two weeks with a supervisor. The supervisor needs to be a qualified professional with experience of working with children and a good knowledge of confidentiality, safeguarding and child welfare issues. A background in the psychological therapies, or specific training in CBT, is a useful but not essential attribute for the group facilitators – so too is an experience of facilitating groups and an awareness of the implications of therapeutic work with children. Having said this, most professionals who facilitate the Cool Connections Programme will adapt the material to their own personal style and theoretical framework.

It is often helpful if the group is facilitated by two people. A qualified person might work, for example, with a teaching assistant based within the school. This helps provide the children with a supportive link person whom they see on a regular basis outside the group, and encourages positive communication and relationships with teaching staff.

AIMS OF THE PROGRAMME

The aims of the programme are to:

- assist children and young people to develop life skills to be able to cope effectively with difficult or anxiety-provoking situations

- normalise the emotional state of anxiety

- build emotional resilience and problem-solving abilities

- encourage peer learning and build peer support networks

- promote self-confidence in dealing with difficult or anxiety-provoking situations

- prevent anxiety and depression in children and young people

- enable children and young people to mix with others and have fun and positive experiences.

EVIDENCE OF EFFECTIVENESS

The Cool Connections Programme has been successfully used in a large number of schools. It has also been run as an after-school group for children of different ages and as a family group programme where parents and children work together with other families. Feedback has been extremely positive from parents, carers, teachers and all participants.

From the large number of individuals who have now taken part, outcome measures have also shown increases in children's coping skills, resilience and self-esteem. Participants have also reported the programme to be fun, helpful and informative.

As the author of the programme, I am frequently contacted by parents, carers and professionals from around the world providing positive feedback after running the programme and requesting further information and additional material. Consequently, this second edition of the programme provides further skills and techniques I have developed since the book was first published.

STRUCTURE OF THE PROGRAMME

The 13 sessions include a mixture of fun games, educational material, therapeutic content and strategies. Participants will be involved in written exercises, discussion, role play, games, puppet work and art activities. They are encouraged to be creative in completing all the exercises and, where possible, interact, share experiences and work with each other in a way that helps normalise their experiences and increases social skills and confidence.

The first two sessions aim to help children get to know each other, build rapport with the facilitators and develop some basic coping resources. Sessions 3–6 help socialise the children to the cognitive model and increase awareness and ability to help children label their thoughts, feelings, body signals and actions. Sessions 7–10 further educate the children and provide strategies to help with the symptoms of anxiety and depression, for example by cognitive restructuring, problem-solving, goal setting, breaking problems down into small steps (building a hierarchy), and using visualisation techniques. In addition to the new material in Session 2, the final part of the book (Sessions 11–13) contains new information which has been included to enhance the Cool Connections Programme and bring it up to date. These sessions include information and exercises related to mindfulness and compassion, which are now an integral part of most CBT practices. These additional sessions also provide further techniques and skills including seeing things from a different perspective, problem-solving, and validating feelings.

Each session in the programme follows the same framework as a cognitive behavioural therapy session:

- Agenda setting

- Home activity review

- Session content, including new material

- Home activity setting.

The Cool Connections Programme sessions generally move at quite a rapid pace and a lot of information and activities are covered in a short space of time. The exercises within each session are generally based on a single theme which is then presented in a range of different ways. It is not necessary, therefore, to complete every exercise in each session. Guidance as to which exercises are most important is provided in 'Agenda and tips for running the session', which is to be found at the start of each session. Depending on the facilitator's timeframe and/or client group, it is fine to be flexible with regard to which of the other exercises are included or left out. Equally, the facilitator may wish to incorporate their own material alongside that provided in each session. There are no hard and fast rules about this. It is fine to adapt the programme to suit individual styles, preferences and group needs.

In keeping with CBT protocol, the group facilitator should aim to work in collaboration with the children and young people wherever possible. A scientific, evidence-based approach to problem-solving is recommended.

RECRUITMENT

Some of the groups we have run have contained children who have been specifically referred by parents or teaching staff. However, the best results have been generated when participants volunteer themselves for the programme. The way this works is that an assembly is held informing children in the school about the programme and inviting them to take part. Those interested are invited to complete a simple questionnaire (similar to the 'Feeling worried' exercise in Session 1), giving their name and reason for wishing to take part. Following consultation with school staff, a group is then chosen. It is interesting to note that most children who volunteer themselves for the group programme are the same children many school staff identify as children 'in need'. While in some clinical settings the volunteering approach may be impractical, encouraging children to volunteer themselves greatly enhances motivation, compliance and rapport building within the group.

In terms of group size, I have experimented with large groups of up to 14 children and smaller groups with as few as four children. From my experience, single-sex groups with between six and eight children of a similar age work best with older children, though this may not be so crucial with younger children.

I have facilitated groups during school time and after school, and had groups that included both parents and children together. In the latter case, the children and parents reported benefiting from the programme.

THE SETTING

The environment for running the programme will depend on the facilities available. Teachers, for example, may prefer children to sit behind desks, while healthcare workers may prefer a circle. Obviously, an environment conducive to learning is best achieved with a spacious, quiet room and a pleasant view. However, this is often not possible, and facilitators will need to make the best of available resources. Very successful programmes can be run with limited resources and difficult working environments.

SUPPORT MATERIAL

Each child in the group should have their own workbook, created from the worksheets contained in this book (which can be photocopied or downloaded from https://library. jkp.com/redeem using the code CEAKAXE). We have experimented by giving children complete workbooks at the start of the programme and also by providing children with A4-style ring-binders where they add a session each week. With the complete workbook, children tend to read ahead instead of focusing on the session in hand. The session-by-session approach works well and enables the facilitator to add or adapt material along the way. Some children like to add their home activity assignments to their folder as they are completed.

TIME PLANNING

The more time given to each session, the more the children will benefit. However, in many schools or organisations, time will be limited. For example, many of the sessions I have run in schools have been restricted to one hour, which is usually the equivalent of one lesson in the school timetable. Although it is possible to run one session within this one-hour timeframe, an hour-and-a-half with a short break is preferable. This provides time to reflect on the previous week's home activity assignments, complete all the exercises and games in the programme, and discuss forthcoming home activity assignments. Additional material (videos, games, etc.) can also be included if required within this longer timeframe. At the start of each session I have provided guidelines for 'short' sessions only one hour in duration and 'long' sessions lasting up to an hour-and-a-half.

HOMEWORK

In line with cognitive behavioural theory, a home activity is given after each session and briefly reviewed with the children at the beginning of the following session. Two different home activities are provided for some sessions. Here the group facilitator can either choose one home activity or give the children both and let them choose which to complete. An enthusiastic group may choose to complete both. Unlike school homework, home activities are voluntary and the children complete them only if they choose to do so. However, it can be explained that they will get more from the programme if they do complete the extra work. In some groups, I have offered a small reward for completing home activities to aid motivation, but this is not essential and is at the discretion of the facilitators.

The home activities are generally linked in some way to the content of that day's session. Most of the activities are intended to be fun and increase children's awareness of the relationship between their thoughts, feelings, body signals and actions (cognitive model). Research suggests that it is through this awareness that change can begin to take place. Children can write home activity feedback on the pages provided (see pages 34–35) at the facilitator's discretion.

Following each session, group leaders are encouraged to meet and reflect on each individual child and on the session as a whole.

DIFFICULTIES IN THE GROUP

Group facilitators, and organisations such as schools or child and adolescent mental health services, will have their own protocols for resolving difficulties that can present when working with groups of children. Facilitators will realise that some parts of the programme may require more skilled facilitation than others. For example, some exercises can be very upsetting for some children. If the distress is not addressed within the group, this can lead to feelings of vulnerability and distrust.

The aim of Cool Connections is to help children cope with feelings of discomfort, and they are therefore encouraged to talk openly about their feelings. At times, children may become quite upset and tearful in session. This can be viewed as a good thing as it suggests that the children are finding the group environment a safe place. However, there is little time allocated within each session to accommodate these feelings. Children's upset feelings need to be validated and empathy offered from within the group, at the same time acknowledging the possible impact on other group members. Children can choose whether to stay within the group for the session or discuss the issue with an appropriate adult on a one-to-one basis outside the group. One of the facilitators can escort a child out of the group if required. In my experience, children most frequently become upset during feedback at the beginning of the session.

CONFIDENTIALITY

In Session 1 the children are informed about confidentiality. At any point in the programme, if a child or parent raises issues regarding the safety of themselves or others (abuse, self-harm, drug-taking, etc.), facilitators are advised to record the information given and follow the child safeguarding procedures within their organisation. It is important that children feel safe in the group or they are unlikely to share information. Children's confidentiality should be respected at all times throughout the programme. Any breach of confidentiality can be addressed openly with the group in the next session. Where appropriate, this can be discussed without naming the individuals involved.

UNDERLYING PRINCIPLES OF CBT

CBT involves development of a shared understanding or formulation of a client's problems. This understanding should inform both therapist and client regarding treatment. Unless each child is given a comprehensive cognitive behavioural assessment prior to undertaking the Cool Connections Programme, individual formulations are difficult to achieve. Consequently, this programme is based on a cognitive behavioural 'approach' which should not be compared with CBT treatment with a trained therapist. However, the material in this programme can be used both in conjunction with CBT treatment and as a useful resource for therapists working with children.

CBT encourages exploration of different ways of thinking, and therapists are encouraged to be non-judgemental in response to the children's thoughts and feelings. There are no right or wrong answers in this programme, although some ways of thinking may be more useful in certain situations than others. The programme aims to increase children's awareness of thoughts, feelings, body signals and actions. It is suggested that through this awareness change can be initiated. Although it is in the nature of young children to think in polarised (black and white) ways, the programme is intended to encourage broader and more flexible thinking (looking for shades of grey) that promotes more acceptance and compassion towards the self and others and consequently a reduction in anxiety and stress levels.

THE COOL CONNECTIONS PROGRAMME
AND THE NATIONAL CURRICULUM

Within the UK the Cool Connections Programme is closely linked with the National Curriculum, especially in relation to PSHE (personal, social and health education) guidelines at Key Stage 2 (7–11 years) and 3 (11–14 years). Links with Key Stage 2 targets are listed below:

- To talk and write about their opinions and explain their views on issues that affect themselves and society.

- To recognise their worth as individuals by identifying positive things about themselves and their achievements, seeing their mistakes, making amendments and setting personal goals.

- To face new challenges positively by collecting information, looking for help, making responsible choices and taking action.

- To see how their actions affect themselves and others, to care about other people's feelings and to try to see things from others' points of view.

- To learn where and how individuals, families and groups can get help and support.

- To reflect on spiritual, moral, social and cultural issues using imagination to understand other people's experiences.

- To resolve differences by looking at alternatives, making decisions and explaining choices.

- To understand what makes a healthy lifestyle, including the benefits of exercise and healthy eating, what affects mental health and how to make informed choices.

- To feel positive about themselves (for example, by producing personal diaries, profiles and portfolios of achievements, by having opportunities to show what they can do and how much responsibility they can take).

Links between the Cool Connections Programme and Key Stage 3 targets, in addition to the above, also include:

- To be able to recognise how others see them and be able to give and receive constructive feedback and praise.

- To understand how to keep healthy.

- To see that good relationships and an appropriate balance between work, leisure and exercise can promote physical and mental health.

- To understand how to empathise with people different from themselves.

- To communicate confidently with peers and adults.

In February 2019, the UK government set out new plans for pupils of all ages to be taught a new subject with a focus on promoting the positive link between physical and mental health from September 2020. The subject will be universal from September 2020 to ensure school prepares pupils for the modern world. The subject material will help primary school pupils learn that mental well-being is a normal part of daily life and why simple self-care, like getting enough sleep and spending time outdoors and with friends, is important. The guidelines state that secondary school pupils should know:

- how to talk about their emotions accurately and sensitively, using appropriate vocabulary

- that happiness is linked to being connected to others

- how to recognise the early signs of mental well-being concerns

- common types of mental ill-health (e.g. anxiety and depression)

- how to critically evaluate when something they do or are involved in has a positive or negative effect on their own or others' mental health

- the benefits and importance of physical exercise, time outdoors, community participation and voluntary and service-based activities on mental well-being and happiness.

The Cool Connections Programme is closely linked with these plans to teach pupils about emotional well-being because it offers a way of encouraging self-esteem, resilience and well-being to young people using CBT approaches. This includes teaching about making good decisions, simple self-care techniques and the skills needed to learn self-control and to regulate emotions.

One Suffolk headteacher I met while running Cool Connections in schools had this to say about the new curriculum plans:

> Using CBT approaches has been invaluable in supporting and empowering children in our school. The impact has been vast; we have seen children's resilience increase and their self-esteem grow, alongside a reduction in anxiety and low mood. The modern world is full of challenges, and CBT has been essential in helping our children identify and face the challenges with a growing confidence. With the new Relationships and Health education becoming compulsory in 2020, Cool Connections is an essential resource for teaching about good mental health. (Amy Arnold, Headteacher, September 2019)

IMPORTANCE OF EARLY INTERVENTION AND PREVENTION PROGRAMMES

There is increasing concern about well-being and mental health in young people. It is considered that children today are facing more stressful conditions than older generations, including increasing competition for jobs, issues of self-identity and confidence driven by more widespread use of social media and the rising costs of housing and higher education. Early intervention has now become a public policy approach to identify and support children and their families and prevent problems developing later in life, such as poor physical and mental health, low educational attainment, crime and anti-social behaviour.

The number of referrals by schools in England seeking mental health treatment for pupils has also risen by more than one third with more than half (55%) of referrals over this period coming from primary schools (NSPCC 2018). Consequently, there is now a government policy to improve young people's mental health that includes commitments set out in the NHS Long Term Plan. Evidence also suggests that most adult mental health disorders start in childhood, with half of adult mental illness starting by the age of 14. Consequently, 'Prevention and early support is vital in meeting the needs of young people. Therefore, early intervention should be given as soon as a problem emerges, at any stage in a child or young person's life' (Department for Education 2018).

The Early Intervention Foundation (2019) also champions the use of effective early intervention to improve the lives of children and young people, stating that:

> The wellbeing and mental health of a child or young person supports positive outcomes in other areas, such as performance at school or behaviour at home. Early intervention can help to build up the social and emotional skills which are so essential for learning and life, support future good mental health, and discourage risky behaviour such as smoking and substance abuse.

Early anxiety intervention programmes including Cool Connections have been shown to reduce the number of children and young people developing anxiety disorders (Morgan, Rapee and Bayer 2016). Furthermore, such programmes are cost effective, in a group-based approach reducing the cost of future professional services, as well as targeting a number of individuals simultaneously over a short period of time. In short, effective early intervention programmes represent a significant opportunity to prevent a great deal of suffering for individuals and their families.

REFERENCES

Morgan, A.J., Rapee, R.M. and Bayer, J.K. (2016) Prevention and Early Intervention of Anxiety Problems in Young Children: A Pilot Evaluation of Cool Little Kids Online. Available at www.ncbi.nlm.nih.gov/pubmed/30135796#.

NSPCC (2018) Early Help (or Early Intervention). Available at https://learning.nspcc.org.uk/safeguarding-child-protection/early-help-early-intervention.

The Early Intervention Foundation (2019) www.eif.org.uk.

Cognitive Behavioural Therapy

The Cool Connections Programme is rooted in the theory of cognitive behavioural therapy (CBT). This section provides a brief summary of the theory and principles of the approach.

Cognitive behavioural therapy emerged in the 1950s and is considered to have evolved from the ideas of Pavlov and Skinner (Salkovskis 1996). The approach is generally associated with the work of Albert Ellis and Aaron Beck that dates back to the early 1970s. The model for CBT arose from Beck's cognitive therapy for depression in the 1960s when he proposed that depressed people are prone to thinking in a distorted way and that they typically have a negative view of themselves, the world and other people (Tarrier 2006). In the 1980s, the cognitive therapists joined forces with behavioural therapists to help challenge people's inaccurate beliefs. The two therapies merged to form the backbone of the CBT approach.

The therapy is a short-term structured approach that involves collaboration between the individual with the problem and the therapist to achieve certain goals. Unlike psychoanalytical psychotherapy, CBT is an evidence-based approach that aims to resolve current problems rather than drawing on assumptions made by the therapist commonly relating to past (unresolved) conflicts. CBT focuses on what the problem is now, what is maintaining it and what can be done to alleviate it (Persons 1989). In CBT, the therapist is considered to work with individuals to help them identify thoughts, feelings and behaviours associated with their problems. Clients are also encouraged to explore different ways of thinking and to consider alternative interpretations of their beliefs. It is further suggested that when clients have developed these skills they can also learn new behaviours and problem-solving strategies with which to reinterpret their thoughts, feelings and behaviours in more rational ways.

There is growing interest in the use of CBT with children and young people. This interest has been encouraged by a number of reviews which conclude that CBT and its variants have been found effective in several childhood and adolescent mental health conditions. A review of the evidence of CBT with children suggests substantial support for CBT as an effective and appropriate first-line treatment for youth with anxiety disorders (Higa-McMillan 2016). 'CBT can be used as an effective treatment for many of the childhood and adolescent mental health conditions provided the familial, cultural, and compatibility perspectives are appropriately considered' (Hadler and Mahato 2019, p.281).

CBT in this age group is seen as an intervention that aims to promote emotional and behavioural change by teaching children to alter their thoughts and thought processes in an overt, active and problem-solving manner. In Ridgeway and Manning's (2018) conceptualisation of the model they suggest children may be helped to identify distorted processing and be guided towards modifying their distorted thinking. Friedberg and McClure (2002) echo this, stating that anxieties, fears and worries are commonplace childhood occurrences. They report that, according to the cognitive model, five spheres of functioning change when children are anxious: physiological, mood, behavioural, cognitive and interpersonal. It has been suggested that treatment for childhood anxieties generally focuses on quietening down distressing symptoms by providing increased coping skills (Semple and Lee 2011):

> CBT is the current 'wonder' treatment and in guidelines published by the National Institute for Clinical Excellence (NICE), CBT has been recommended as the treatment of choice for a number of conditions ranging from post-traumatic stress disorder to depression. At this point in time CBT has established itself as the therapy for children most strongly backed by scientific evidence although the evidence base is still quite limited. (Stallard 2007)

Although the literature on the treatment of children and adolescents with CBT is far less extensive than that for adults, a number of studies have confirmed the short-term efficacy and safety of treatments for anxiety and depression in young people. A study supported by the National Alliance on Mental Illness (2007) comparing different types of psychotherapy for major depression in children found that CBT led to remission in nearly 65 per cent of cases, a higher rate than that following either supportive therapy or family therapy. CBT also resulted in a more rapid treatment response. Results are higher in relation to children with anxiety. Children with anxiety are reported to have approximately a 70–80 per cent response rate with CBT, and the gains are maintained over time.

Until recently it has been suggested that young children are unlikely to understand cognitive concepts and therefore will not benefit from CBT. Consequently, play or systemic family therapy have been considered more appropriate treatments. However, in recent years there has been increasing evidence that CBT may be effective with both children and adolescents. With parental support, children as young as two or three can learn how to use non-anxious self-talk (using puppets or dolls as models) and desensitisation through gradual exposure.

Stallard (2008) proposes that CBT approaches with young people need to be modified to coincide with the individual's developmental stage and cognitive abilities. It is suggested that it is the way the CBT material is presented that needs to change as opposed to the approach being inappropriate. He notes that you would not expect to achieve positive outcomes with children when applying unadapted adult tools. This is echoed by Ridgeway and Manning (2018) who suggest that CBT therapy with children needs to be adapted from the adult model to suit the age of the individual. The CBT approach is considered to help children challenge their thoughts and understanding of situations, rather than accepting their thoughts as the truth. CBT encourages children to generate more realistic versions of situations and their ability to cope with them. Ready with a new mindset, children then gradually face difficult or fearful situations, breaking the challenges down into small, manageable steps. Over time, children are able to tap more quickly into non-anxious interpretations of situations, and in some cases understand that avoidance of feared situations can help maintain their difficulties.

With an increasing number of studies in recent years providing empirical evidence of the effectiveness of CBT with children, both on an individual basis and in groups, there is a strong case for using CBT to achieve the kinds of long-term improvements in children and young people described in this summary. Stallard reflects this, stating: 'Effectiveness needs to be substantiated and there is a national need to improve the availability and practice of CBT with children and young people' (Stallard 2007).

REFERENCES

Friedberg, R.D. and McClure, J.M. (2002) *Clinical Practice of Cognitive Therapy with Children and Adolescents: The Nuts and Bolts.* New York, NY: Guilford Press.

Hadler, S. and Mahato, A.K. (2019) 'Cognitive behavior therapy for children and adolescents: Challenges and gaps in practice.' *Indian Journal of Psychological Medicine*, 41, 3, 279–283.

Higa-McMillan, C. (2016) 'Evidence base update: 50 years of research on treatment for child and adolescent anxiety.' *Journal of Clinical Child and Adolescent Psychology*, 45, 2, 91–113.

National Alliance on Mental Illness (2007) Helpline Facts Sheet: Children and Adolescent OCD. Accessed on 11/01/08 at www.nami.org/learn-more/mental-health-conditions/obsessive-compulsive-disorder.

Persons, J.B. (1989) *Cognitive Therapy in Practice: A Case Formulation Approach.* New York, NY: W.W. Norton & Company.

Ridgeway, N. and Manning, J. (2018) *CBT Worksheet for Kids – OCD: A CBT Worksheets Book for CBT Therapists, CBT Therapists in Training & Trainee Clinical Psychologists.* Bury St Edmunds: West Suffolk CBT Services.

Salkovskis, P.M. (1996) *Frontiers of Cognitive Therapy.* New York, NY: Guilford Press.

Semple, R.J. and Lee, J. (2011) *A Manual for Treating Childhood Anxiety: Mindfulness-Based Cognitive Therapy for Anxious Children.* Oakland, CA: New Harbinger Publications.

Stallard, P. (2007) Expert's Concerns about Child Mental Health Services. Accessed on 11/01/08 at www.bath.ac.uk/news/2007/4/11/paulstallardlecture.html.

Stallard, P. (2008) *CBT with Children, Adolescents and Families: Anxiety. Cognitive Behaviour Therapy with Children and Young People.* London and New York, NY: Routledge.

Tarrier, N. (ed.) (2006) *Case Formulation in Cognitive Behaviour Therapy: The Treatment of Challenging and Complex Cases.* Oxford: Oxford University Press.

Useful Links and Resources

The programme acknowledges the ideas and inspiration of others who have gone before, including the following:

Alexander, J. (2003) *Bullies, Bigmouths and So-Called Friends*. London: Hodder Children's Books.

Altiero, J. (2007) *No More Stinking Thinking: A Workbook for Teaching Children Positive Thinking*. London and Philadelphia, PA: Jessica Kingsley Publishers.

Azri, S. (2013) *Healthy Mindsets for Super Kids: A Resilience Programme for Children Aged 7–14*. London: Jessica Kingsley Publishers.

Bartkowiak, J. (2010) *NLP for Children (Engaging NLP)*. London: MX Publishing.

Beever, S. (2009) *Happy Kids Happy You: Using NLP to Bring Out the Best in Ourselves and the Children We Care For*. Carmarthen, Wales: Crown House Publishing.

British Association for Behavioural and Cognitive Psychotherapies: www.babcp.com.

Chansky, T.E. (2004) *Freeing Your Child from Anxiety: Powerful, Practical Solutions to Overcome Your Child's Fears, Worries, and Phobias*. New York, NY: Broadway Books.

Collins-Donnelly, K. (2014) *Starving the Anxiety Gremlin for Children Aged 5–9: A Cognitive Behavioural Therapy Workbook on Anxiety Management*. London: Jessica Kingsley Publishers.

Coombes, S., Murray, L. and Abey, K. (2017) *No Worries! Mindful Kids: An Activity Book for Young People Who Sometimes Feel Anxious or Stressed*. London: Studio Press Books.

Freeland, C.A.B. and Toner, J.B. (2016) *What to Do When You Feel Too Shy: A Kid's Guide to Overcoming Social Anxiety*. Washington, DC: Magination Press.

Friedberg, R.D. (2001) *Therapeutic Exercises for Children Workbook: Guided Self-Discovery Using Cognitive-Behavioral Techniques*. Sarasota, FL: Professional Resource Exchange.

Gomez, A.M. (2012) *EMDR Therapy and Adjunct Approaches with Children: Complex Trauma, Attachment, and Dissociation*. New York, NY: Springer Publishing Company.

Huebner, D. (2005) *What to Do When You Worry Too Much: A Kid's Guide to Overcoming Anxiety*. Washington, DC: Magination Press.

Huebner, D. and Matthews, B. (2007) *What to Do When Your Brain Gets Stuck: A Kid's Guide to Overcoming OCD*. Washington, DC: Magination Press.

Huebner, D. and Matthews, B. (2009) *What to Do When Bad Habits Take Hold: A Kid's Guide to Overcoming Nail Biting and More*. Washington, DC: Magination Press.

Hutt, R. (2019) *Feel Better: CBT Workbook for Teens: Essential Skills and Activities to Help You Manage Moods, Boost Self-Esteem, and Conquer Anxiety*. Emeryville, CA: Althea Press.

Kendall, P.C. and Hedtke, K.A. (2006) *The Coping Cat Workbook, Second Edition*. Ardmore, PA: Workbook Publishing.

Kendall, P.C. and MacDonald, J.P. (1993) 'Cognition in the Psychopathology of Youth and Implications for Treatment.' In K.S. Dobson and P.C. Kendall (eds) *Psychopathology and Cognition* (pp.387–427). San Diego, CA: Academic Press.

Lucado, M. (2011) *Max Lucado's You Are Special and 3 Other Stories: A Children's Treasury Box Set*. Nashville, TN: Tommy Nelson Publishers.

Mall, M. and Stringer, B. (2002) *Understanding Behaviour: Psychology for Parents and Teachers Working with Family Groups*. Birmingham: Questions Publishing Company.

Manning, J. and Ridgeway, N. (2018) *Joe Goes to OCD School: A CBT Book for Kids Who Are Struggling with OCD*. Bury St Edmunds: West Suffolk CBT Services.

McCauley, E. *et al.* (2016) *Behavioral Activation with Adolescents: A Clinician's Guide*. New York, NY: Guilford Press.

Micco, J.A. (2017) *The Worry Workbook for Teens: Effective CBT Strategies to Break the Cycle of Chronic Worry and Anxiety*. Canada: Instant Help Books.

Moser, A.J. (1988) *Don't Pop Your Cork on Mondays! The Children's Anti-Stress Book*. Kansas City, MO: Landmark Editions.

Phifer, L. *et al.* (2017) *CBT Toolbox for Children and Adolescents: Over 220 Worksheets & Exercises for Trauma, ADHD, Autism, Anxiety, Depression & Conduct Disorders*. Eau Claire, WI: PESI Publishing & Media.

Rapee, R.M., Spence, S.H., Cobham, V. and Wignall, A. (2000) *Helping Your Anxious Child: A Step-by-Step Guide for Parents*. Oakland, CA: New Harbinger Publications.

Rapee, R.M., Wignall, A., Hudson, J.L. and Schniering, C.A. (2000) *Treating Anxious Children and Adolescents: An Evidence-Based Approach*. Oakland, CA: New Harbinger Publications.

Stallard, P. (2018) *Think Good Feel Good: A Cognitive Behaviour Therapy Workbook for Children*. Chichester: John Wiley & Sons.

Stark, K. and Kendall, P.C. (1996) *Treating Depressed Children: Therapist Manual for 'Taking Action'*. Ardmore, PA: Workbook Publishing.

Stringer, B. and Mall, M. (1999) *A Solution Focused Approach to Anger Management with Children*. Birmingham: Questions Publishing Company.

PRE-GROUP MATERIAL

PRE-GROUP MATERIAL CONTENTS

Individual recording sheet

Facilitators are encouraged to record information following sessions. They may find this a useful format for recording information about individuals.

Assessment tool: What RU like?

For those facilitators able to offer a one-to-one session to children before the programme begins. This tool aims to provide some background information and help build rapport between children and the facilitators before the group begins.

Cool Connections Programme self-referral form

A useful form that children can complete themselves to take part in the programme (following a school assembly for example).

Home activity feedback

Some children or facilitators may find it useful to record what individual children have learned from their home activities each week.

> The worksheets contained in this book can be photocopied or downloaded from https://library.jkp.com/redeem using the code CEAKAXE

Individual recording sheet

Name: **Group facilitator(s):**

Date/session number	Comments

Date/session number	Comments

Date/session number	Comments

Date/session number	Comments

Date/session number	Comments

Date/session number	Comments

Date/session number	Comments

Date/session number	Comments

Date/session number	Comments

Date/session number	Comments

Assessment tool: What RU like?

My favourite things are...	
My friends say I am...	
My mum is...	
My dad is...	
My school is...	
I feel angry about...	
The things I'm sad about are...	
The things I'm frightened of are...	
I don't like...	
My secret is...	
If I had a magic wand I would...	
If I could ask one question without upsetting anyone I would ask...	

Adapted from Herbert, M. (1991) *Clinical Child Psychology: Social Learning, Development and Behaviour*. Chichester: Wiley.

Cool Connections Programme self-referral form

We are running a group to help children cope with their feelings. The group will involve some fun games, acting, stories, art work and learning more about feelings. If you want to join the group, complete the information below.

What is your name?

. . . .

How often do you worry or feel sad about things? Tick the box which best describes you.

Never		Sometimes		Every day	

Where do you feel most sad or worried? Tick the box which best describes you.

Never		Sometimes		Every day	

Why do you think you should be included in the Cool Connections Programme?

. . . .

. . . .

. . . .

Home activity feedback

What did you learn or notice from your homework this week?

1.

2.

3.

4.

5.

6.

7.

8.

9.

10.

SESSIONS

SESSION 1: GETTING TO KNOW EACH OTHER

Aims and objectives

- Enable group members to get to know each other.

- Agree some group rules.

- Begin learning about feelings and make some goals.

- Begin sharing feelings with other members of the group.

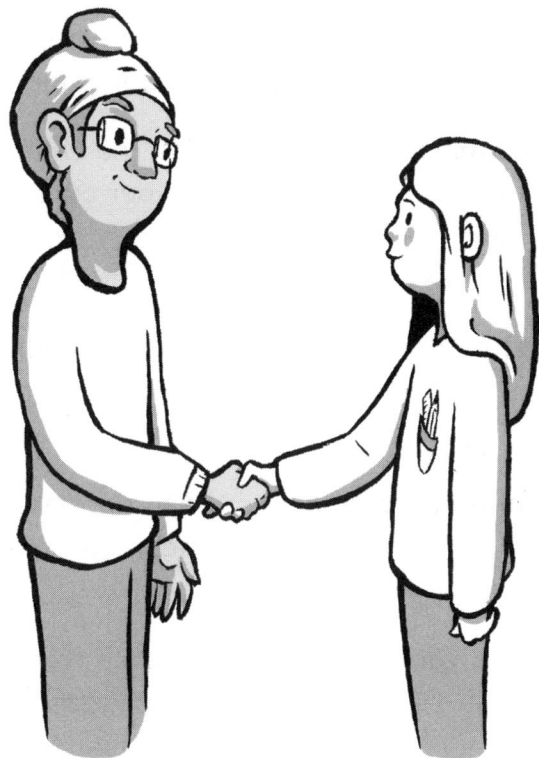

- Have fun.

Materials

Chairs, pencils.

Agenda and tips for running the session

Exercises in bold in the left-hand column should be included in both long and short sessions. Many fun activities and games are included as optional. Despite sometimes being short of time, it is important not to cut all the 'fun' out of the programme or you will lose the children's enthusiasm.

Short session

EXERCISE	COMMENT
Welcome children	Share agenda for session with group.
Meet the gang	There are four characters who feature throughout the programme: Katie, Amir, Jack and Lauren. This exercise introduces the characters to the group.
All change game	This game can be adapted to suit the group. The general aim is to help children relax and get to know each other.
Confidentiality	Important to share this for professional reasons and to develop trust within the group.
Group rules	Give the children a list of the rules (see page 47 or make up your own). The group members can sign and return it for the next session. This is only a guide. Group facilitators may choose to alter or change the rules at their discretion.
Who am I?	Having completed this exercise, ask the children to feed back two bits of information about themselves of their choice. This might include only their name.
Feeling worried	Read the paragraph at the top of the first page and take one or two examples from the children without completing the boxes.
Rate yourself	Children frequently find this difficult. It is better if they can be specific about areas in their life that they hope taking part in the group will help with. Where children have difficulty coming up with things for themselves or identifying their own personal problems, they can be asked questions such as: 'If a friend had the chance to be involved in this programme, what do you think it would help him with?' At this stage in the programme, children can be given the choice whether they share information with the rest of the group or not.

'Flipping your lid'   Some children are very self-conscious about acting (page 54), especially in the first session. This can be overcome by encouraging the children to draw a picture or just talk about a scenario with a friend without acting. This self-consciousness can provide information about some children's anxiety and it can be very helpful to encourage them to work through this. Our experience is that the children's confidence grows as the programme progresses.

Home activity 1a: My family   Children can complete this in any way they choose (stick men are fine). This activity helps the children get to know one another better. It also provides facilitators with more information about an individual's support network. Much can be gained from close observation of the children's drawings, for example who they include or miss out from pictures, and who is close to whom – also facial characteristics. It is important to check out with the children observations taken from drawings rather than jumping to conclusions. Quality of drawings is unimportant but may help facilitators identify personality traits, such as perfectionism.

Home activity 1b: Hopes and dreams   This activity helps children to be specific about their difficulties and their goals and helps them generate some solutions of their own. There is much research suggesting that the clearer you can imagine your dreams for the future, the closer you become to making them reality. The drawings only have to mean something to the children.

The exercise encourages children to visualise their difficulties and how they could be resolved. It could be used in place of the rating scales on pages 53 and 252, compared with pictures drawn at the end of the programme.

Long session

As above but more time can be spent on warm-up games. Group rules can be discussed in session and created by the children. The 'Feeling worried' exercise can be completed in full.

Notes

The most important aspect of this session is to give the children a positive experience and for them to begin to get to know one another. This helps in developing trust and in normalising the children's feelings. It can be very therapeutic to see that other children have worries and problems too. There are a lot of different activities in this first session. You may choose to change the games or activities to suit your timeframe.

Meet the gang

Meet the four characters below. They will be helping you by offering pictures and examples as you work through the Cool Connections Programme.

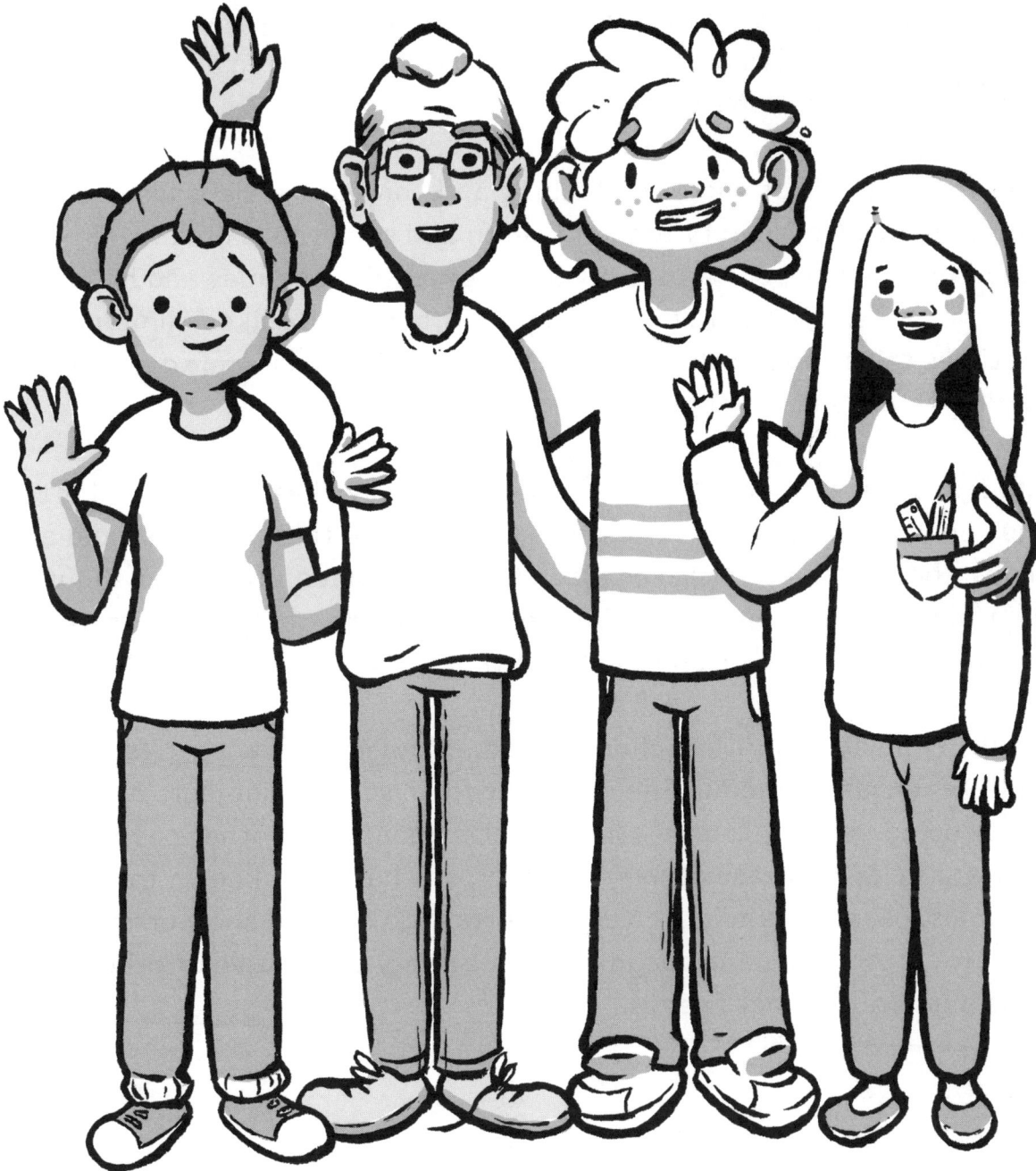

From the pictures and thought bubbles shown in the programme you may assume the following about each of the characters:

Katie: Likes to relax in the sunshine and likes the company of Jack. She tends to opt out of things and does not like sports. Katie can be bossy towards other children and thinks of herself as both fat and ugly. Sometimes when she is with other people she tries to hide her unhappy feelings by wearing a 'happy' mask. Katie can sometimes be bossy towards other children and has a quick temper when things don't go her way.

Amir: Amir really likes snooker, climbing and computers. He is also good at building things. Amir is very fond of Lauren and sometimes dreams of being a superhero. He has poor eyesight which upsets him at times and he is very frightened of snakes and worries about his health. He likes climbing and sometimes talks about other children behind their backs. Amir does not get on well with his teacher at school.

Jack: Fun to be with and good at sports. Especially likes football and often comes up with good ideas. Sometimes at school he thinks he is stupid and worries about making mistakes. Jack's parents often argue and shout at him at home. This often makes him feel angry inside. Jack is very scared of spiders. He can also be mean to Katie at times.

Lauren: Popular with other children and enjoys lots of activities such as diving, tennis and dancing. She is also good at science subjects at school. Despite being popular, Lauren often worries about what other people think of her and tries to please others. However, she has been known to be cruel to animals. Lauren's family are very important to her and she worries about being away from them. Although she can be very supportive of others, she can be a gossip with her friends.

All change game

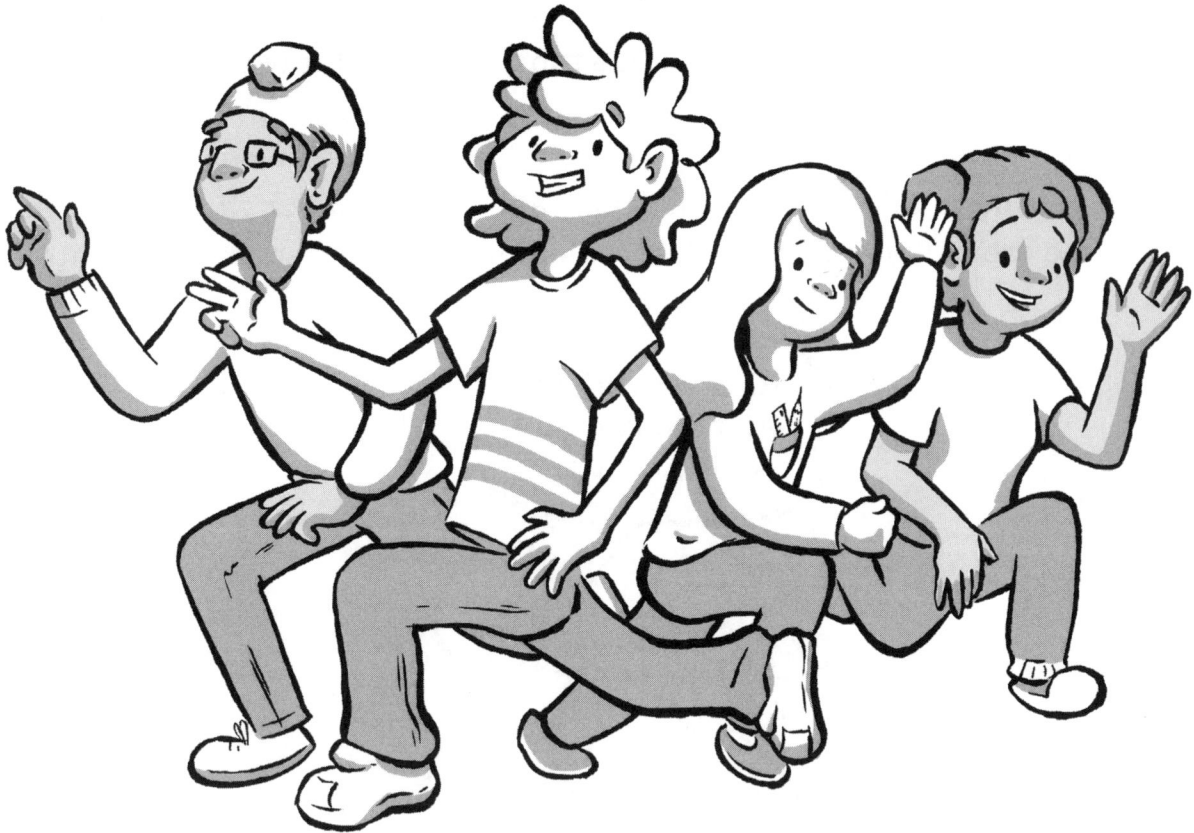

'All change' is an easy game to play. It is a fun way of getting to know other group members and making cool connections with each other. To play the game, group members sit in a circle facing each other on their chairs. The group facilitator shouts 'all change' and everyone swaps seats. After a few turns, one chair is taken away. When everyone has changed chairs the person left in the middle tells the group something about themselves, then shouts 'all change'. The game can be repeated as many times as you like. This game helps you to get to know each other and to learn how people are different.

Confidentiality

'Confidentiality' means that what we talk about in the group is special to the group and we won't tell anyone outside the group about it without asking the group first.

It's OK for you to talk to your own family and friends about what you do and say in the group if you want to, but remember, what others say is private.

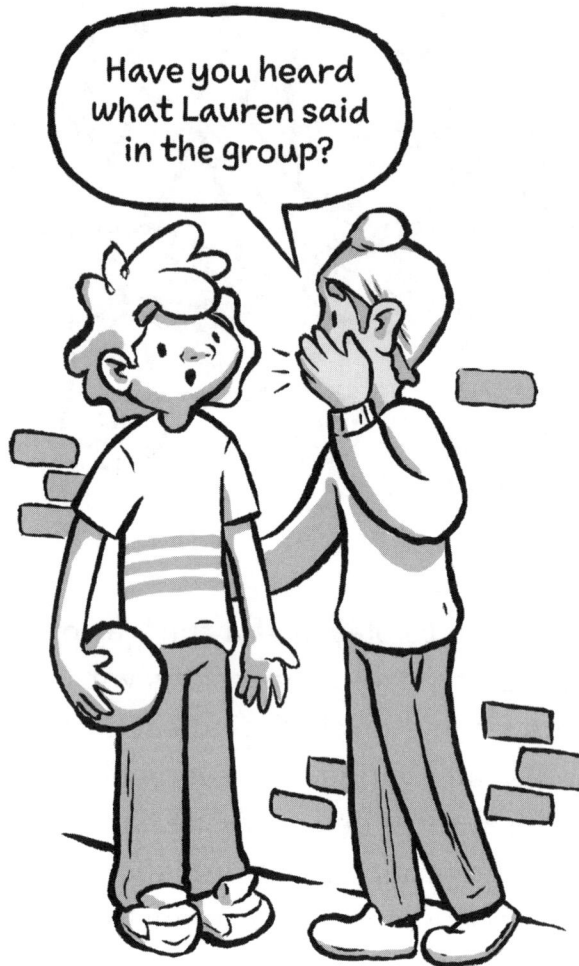

If you tell the group facilitators anything that makes them think that you are not safe outside the group or that you are in danger, they will have to talk to someone outside the group who can help protect you. But they will try to tell you what they are doing and why. The most important thing is that you are safe.

Group rules

Respect each other

It is important that we each try to respect other children in the group and the group facilitators. This involves supporting and listening to each other and taking turns to speak.

Timekeeping

It makes it difficult if you are not on time for the group to start. While it is the responsibility of the group facilitators to ensure groups are organised to start and finish on time, it is your responsibility not to be late.

Personal choice

It is your choice to be in the group. By making this choice you can decide to leave at any time. However, for safety reasons it is important that you let the group facilitators know of your whereabouts at all times. If you are disrupting the group your actions will suggest that you no longer wish to take part and you will be given the choice to either stay and stop disrupting the session or leave the group. If you choose to leave on more than one occasion, you may be asked to leave the group altogether.

Commitment

It is important that if you are to get something out of this group then you are prepared to put something in of yourself. We hope to encourage all of the group to take part in all the activities. However, we will not make anyone do anything. By making the commitment to become part of the group you also commit to doing the home activity work and taking part in all group activities, not just the ones you like.

I agree to keep to the group rules and to stick to the confidentiality agreement

Signature: . . . .

Who am I?

Complete the following sentences about yourself.

My name is:

The people in my family are:

I like to:

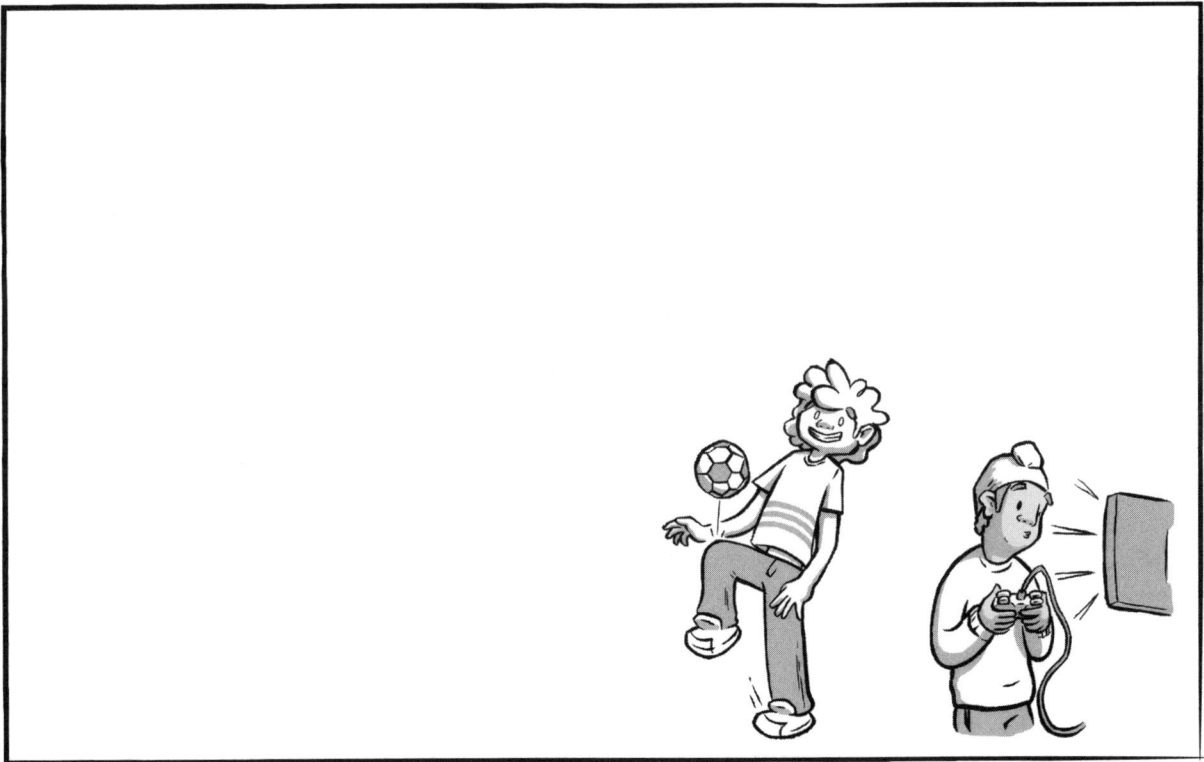

The worst thing in my life is:

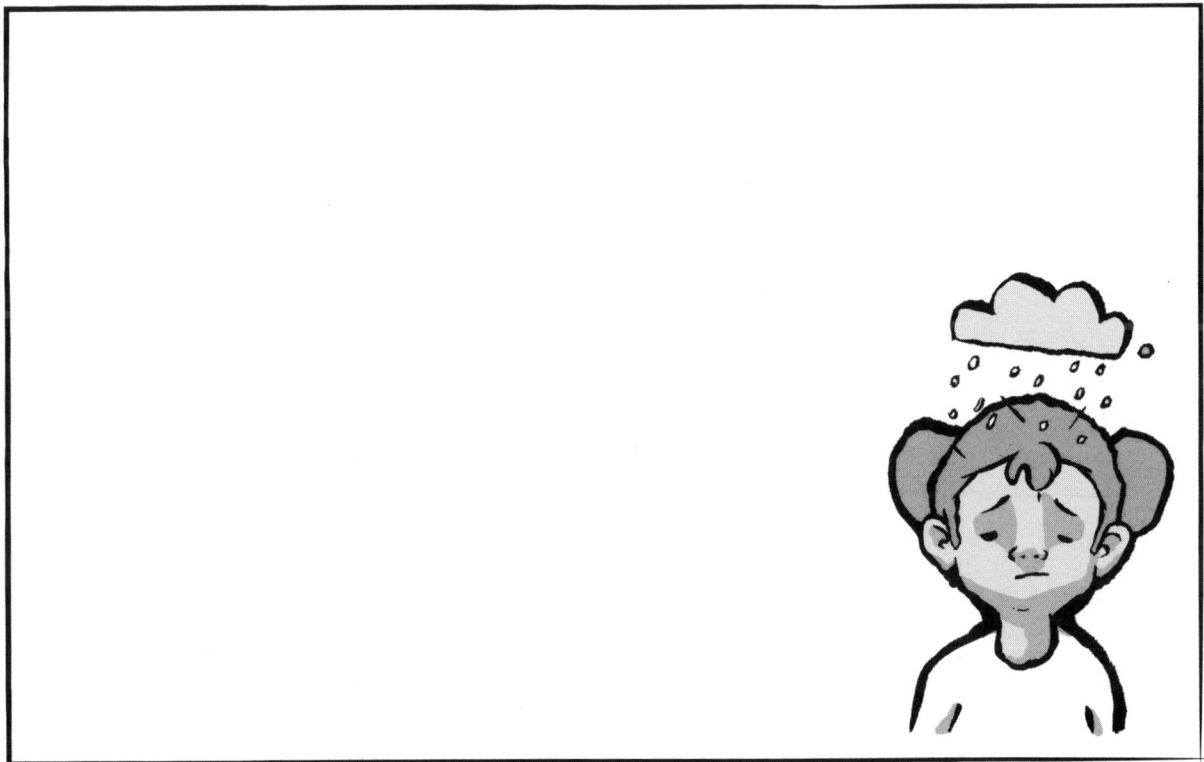

Nice things my friends say about me are:

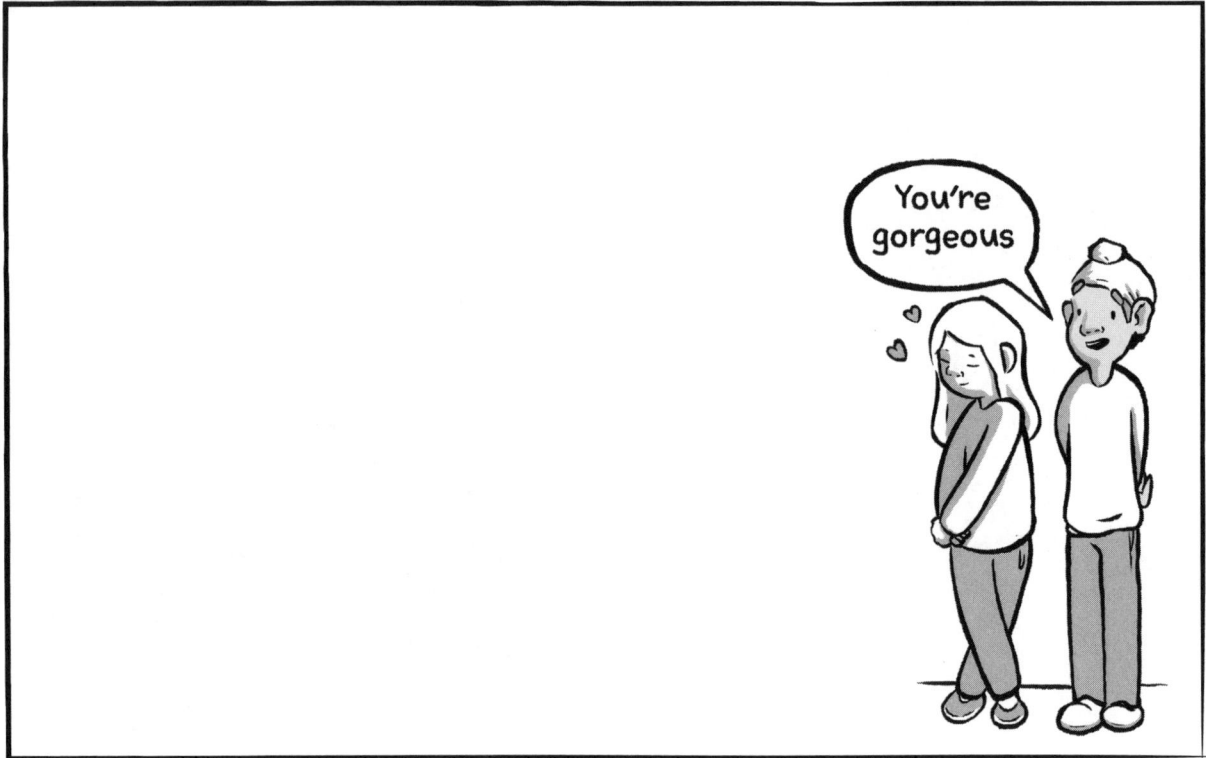

One thing I would like to change about myself is:

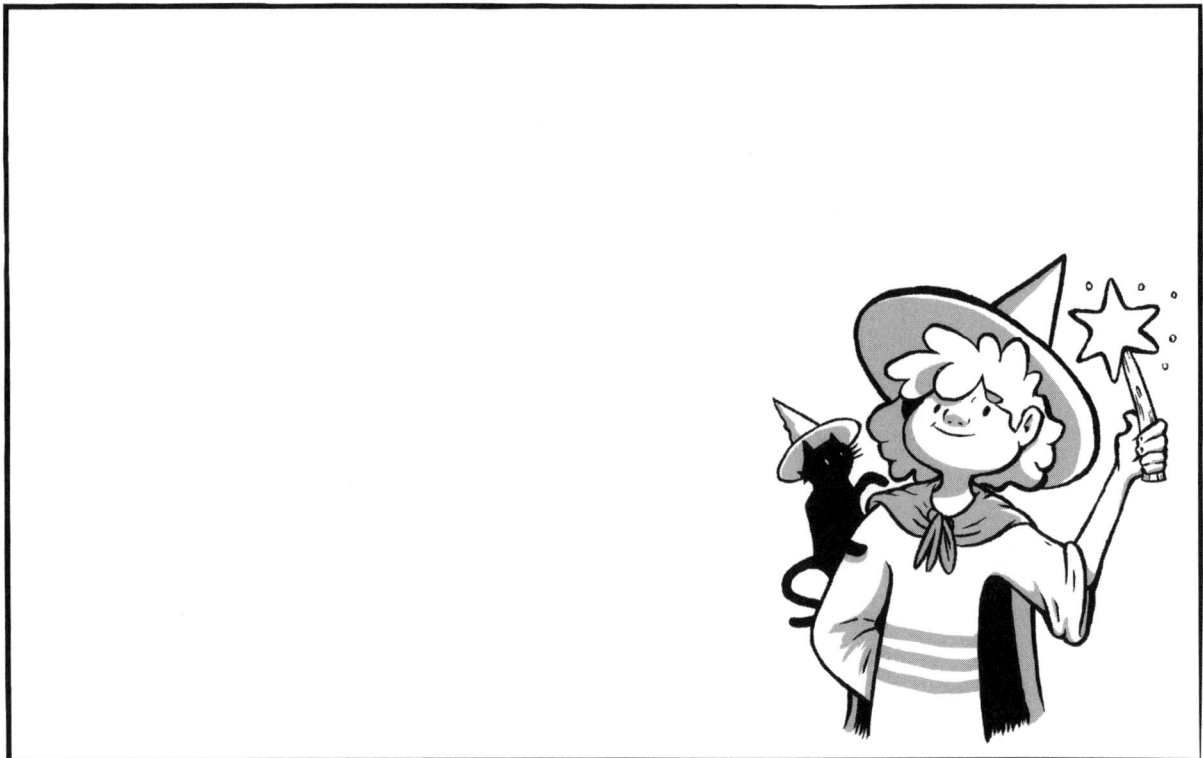

Feeling worried

Everyone has feelings and gets worried sometimes no matter how old or young they are. People get scared about different things too. Some children are scared of animals like snakes or bears, while others worry about things such as the dark or heights. Sometimes children worry about making new friends, going to parties, doing school work or being away from their mums, dads or home. Whatever it is that makes each of us feel worried, being afraid is a feeling everyone has sometimes.

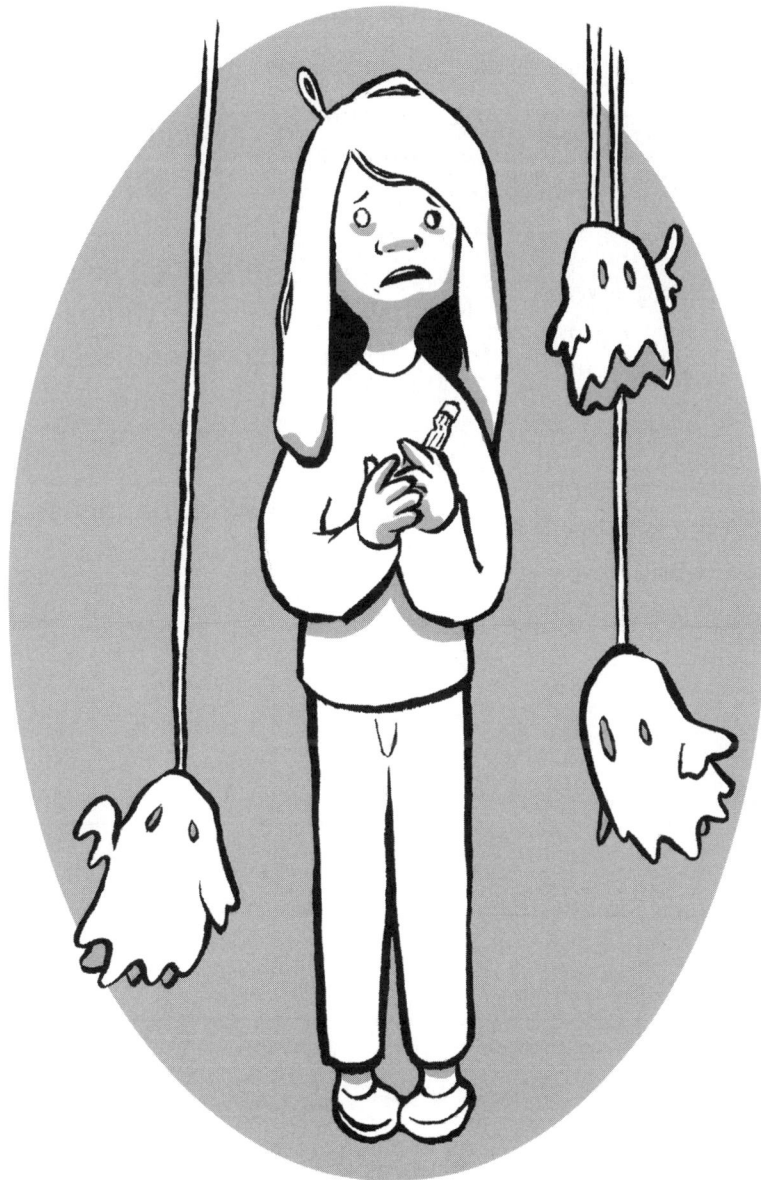

Below are some of the things lots of children worry about. Please tick the boxes which best describe your worries. If there are any things you worry about that are not on the list, write them in the empty spaces at the bottom.

Spiders	Hospitals	Going to school	Snakes	The dark
Arguments at home	Speaking out in class	Keeping my family safe	Germs and dirt	Being told off
Eating in front of other kids	Being sick	Using the telephone	Being bullied	Making mistakes
Scary thoughts I can't get rid of	Being away from mum and dad	Not having many friends	Feeling I have to do things over and over again	Being fat and ugly
Secrets I can't talk about to do with home or school	What other kids think about me	Getting a serious illness like cancer or AIDS	What happens when I die	Being attacked

Rate yourself

Mark a cross on the number you currently feel most represents your life and how you are coping at the moment both in and out of school.

1	2	3	4	5	6	7	8	9	1 0

VERY UPSET   **HAPPY**

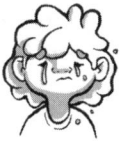

List three things below which you feel most upset about in your life at the moment. Put a cross on the number which best represents how you feel.

Example: I have not got many friends

1	2̶	3	4	5	6	7	8	9	1 0

VERY UPSET   **HAPPY**

1: ....

1	2	3	4	5	6	7	8	9	1 0

VERY UPSET   **HAPPY**

2: ....

1	2	3	4	5	6	7	8	9	1 0

VERY UPSET   **HAPPY**

3: ....

1	2	3	4	5	6	7	8	9	1 0

VERY UPSET   **HAPPY**

Flipping your lid

It happens all the time. People 'flip their lids' when they get worried, upset or lose their cool. This is often caused by something called stress.

Everyone becomes stressed from time to time. It can affect doctors, teachers, dancers, sportsmen, drivers and shop workers too. Mothers and fathers can become stressed when they can't pay the bills, when they have too much work to do, or when there are long queues on the roads or in the supermarkets. Children also can become stressed when they can't understand their school work, when other children pick on them, or when adults don't listen to them.

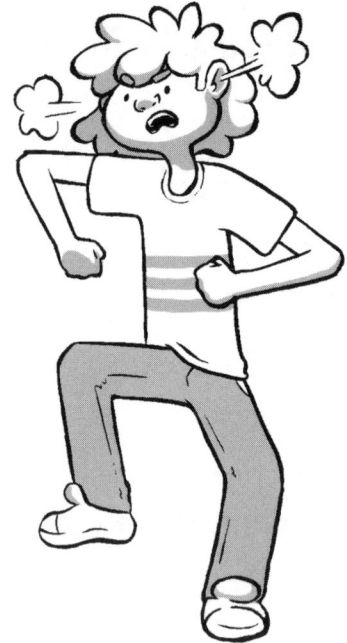

The trouble with stress is that it often gets passed on from one person to another. For example, if business is poor, the boss gets upset with an employee. During lunch, the employee is rude to a waitress. The waitress goes home that night and scolds her children. Finally, the children yell at the cat. But what is the poor cat supposed to do?

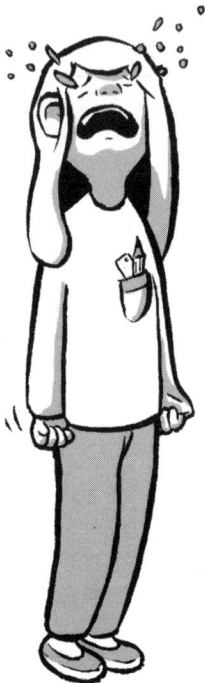

People often behave differently when they are under stress. People can start to shout or act like wild animals. Some people growl and roar like tigers; others go crazy like wild monkeys. Some people even lose control and charge like rhinoceroses breaking up everything in sight. Still others become quiet and hide away like a tortoise in its shell. Some people cry real crocodile tears, while others refuse to face the problem and bury their heads in the sand like ostriches.

In the Cool Connections Programme, we are going to look at some cool ways to cope with those bottled-up feelings which cause stress and can cause people to 'flip their lids'. These feelings include fear, anger, sadness and guilt.

You will learn to become more aware of your thoughts, feelings, body signals and actions. With this information you can learn to recognise your feelings and explore new ways to cope when you feel angry, worried, down or stressed. By learning the 'cool connections' between your thoughts, feelings, body signals and actions, you will become less likely to 'flip your lid' and more likely to 'stay cool'!

Think of a time when you have felt unhappy and stressed. With a friend, act out the scene and show it to the group.

Give a brief description of the scene you acted in the box below.

Home activity 1a: My family

Draw a picture of your family. Include yourself in the picture.

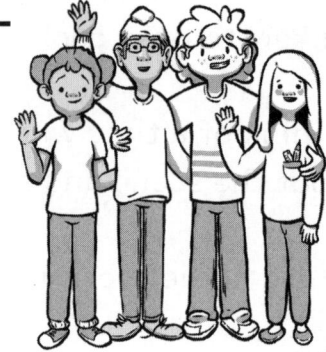

Home activity 1b: Hopes and dreams

On the lines below, list two things you hope the group will help you with:

1. . . . .

. . . .

2. . . . .

. . . .

In the box below, draw one of your main worries or problems.

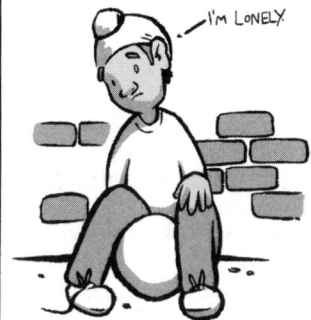

In the box below, draw what your worry or problem would look like 'all better'.

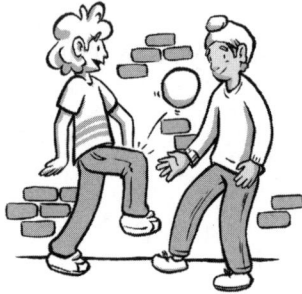

In the box below, draw a way you could get from Box 1 (your problem) to Box 2 (your 'all better').

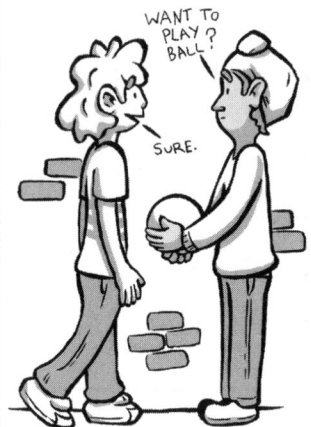

SESSION 2: RESOURCES

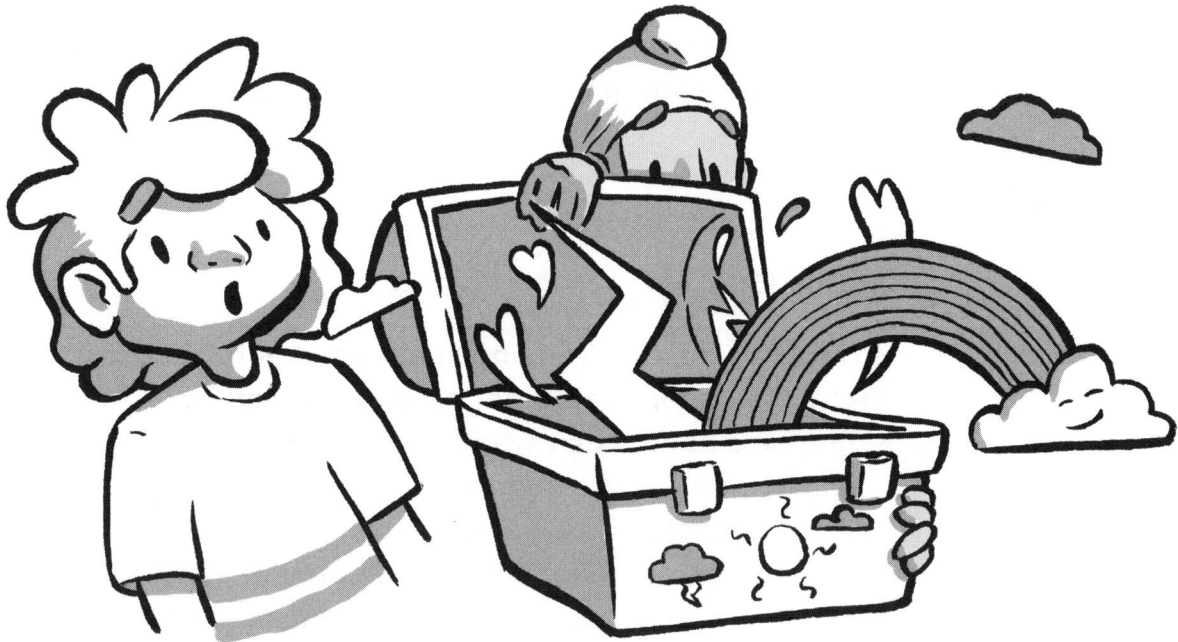

Aims and objectives

- Help individuals in the group begin to regulate their emotions and calm themselves when they feel stressed.

- Identify supportive people in the children's lives.

- Learn to use imagination to overcome difficulties and explore alternative solutions.

- Share different ideas about 'looking after your emotions' with the group.

Materials

Pencils, coloured pens/crayons (optional).

Materials to make a container (small wooden craft boxes, for example) (optional).

Agenda and tips for running the session

Exercises in bold in the left-hand column should be included in both long and short sessions. To save time in short sessions, omit the 'Super special helper' exercise; similar exercises are included in other parts of the programme.

Short session

EXERCISE	COMMENT
Feedback	Welcome the children and share agenda for the session with the group. Gain brief feedback from group members about their week. This feedback needs to be very brief or it can quickly consume the majority of the session. One piece of information from each child is recommended. If children provide upsetting or concerning feedback at this time empathy should be given, and one-to-one time to discuss the issue in detail is recommended following the session.
Review Home activities 1a and 1b	Children briefly show their drawings from Home activities 1a and 1b. It may be interesting to notice which family members are included and any that are left out. Sometimes facilitators will notice things about the children's drawings or hopes and dreams that are relevant to their difficulties. These issues can be discussed within the group at the discretion of facilitators.
Care and compassion	Encourage individuals to read through the text. If group members struggle to identify anyone who is caring from their own lives, they can either make up a character, use a superhero from the TV or ask for support from the group. Children can also think of people they have seen being kind to someone else. The idea is to encourage the children to begin to identify with what caring/nurture looks like and how they can recognise someone with these qualities.

Protective figures and wise figures	Children need to feel safe and protected. Group members may also find it helpful to identify with a wise figure whose wisdom they can draw on if they need help. Again, if children struggle to identify characters from their own life they can make it up or use magical creatures or superheroes.
Calm place	Unfortunately, some children do not have a place of safety or lack the ability to calm themselves down. Developing a calm place helps children begin to find ways of self-soothing and to regulate their emotions. This is an exercise that is used in a number of different therapies. The clearer the picture that group members can create in their imaginations, the more useful the exercise will be. Calm places can be strengthened by encouraging the children to include sounds, smells and emotions within their images.
Cool containers	Children frequently find it useful to put their 'too big' feelings in an imaginary container. This does not need to be a box. It could be a bag, book, time capsule or even somewhere hidden inside a mystical creature. Some group members may choose to make their container or even use it between sessions to write their feelings down on paper to keep safely inside.
Super special helper	Most children have good imaginations. This could be a character that is made up or a friend, pet or creature if they prefer. Children can share their ideas with the group. Some children like to make their super special helper. This can be done with modelling clay, plasticine or wooden spoons and craft materials.
Home activity 2: Resource Figures	Children are encouraged to practise the resources they have developed in Session 2. For homework, the group are encouraged to identify times they have used resources and to monitor outcomes.

Long session

As above but more time can be spent in discussion or sharing ideas within the group. Include the 'Super special helper' exercise if you have time in the longer session.

Notes

The aim of this session is to help the group members develop resources and learn some basic strategies for calming themselves down when they become stressed. If children have these skills in place they will be learning really useful life skills. Group members will also begin to feel safer sharing their feelings without becoming so overwhelmed. Part of building resources is to identify the supportive figures the children already have in their lives. This can include imaginary helpers, pets, animals or the caring/loving qualities of people who are no longer alive, such as great-grandparents.

Care and compassion (nurture)

Compassion means we care about others, treat them with kindness, and feel a strong desire to help those in need. Compassion is also sometimes called empathy. This could be like giving a hug, making a card or saying something kind to help a friend or family member who is feeling sad or upset. It can also look like reaching out to a friend who has been left out, or wanting to do something to help others at home or school, even if you do not know the person. It is also possible to have compassion for animals such as your pets at home. When someone is caring they can be described as a nurture figure. In the box below draw or list people from your life who are caring towards others and can make you feel loved. This can be real people, pets or even made-up characters from books or the TV.

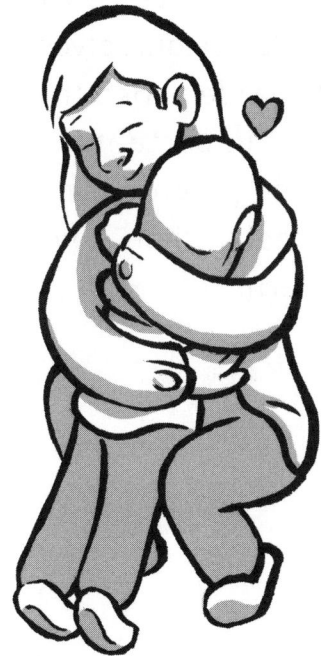

While it is good to care about others, it is also important to become compassionate and caring towards ourselves. This is part of developing self-esteem. When we forgive ourselves, it becomes easier to cope with uncomfortable thoughts and feelings. Some people say that if we do not care for ourselves we may find difficulty caring for others. Psychologists have identified that it is important for everyone to know that they are special and important. Children feel this way when they get love and praise from their parents, kind grown-ups and sometimes their friends. If you do not feel special, then it will be difficult for you to cope with things in school and to learn.

Protective figures

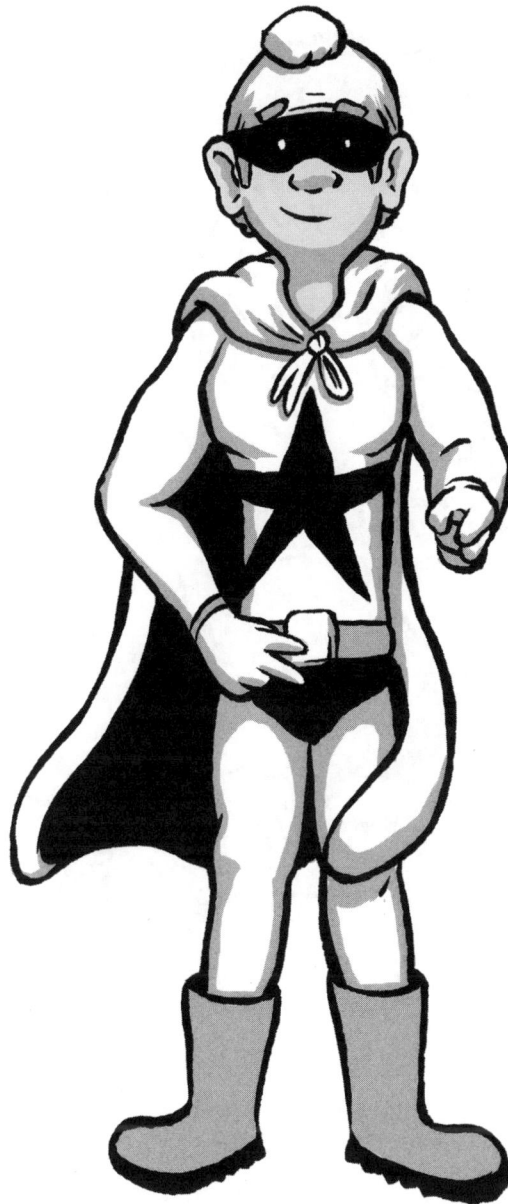

As well as nurture, for our survival, feeling safe and protected is another important area in our lives. Without this, we become stressed and can feel in a state of high alert – just like when a fox sees the hounds or a rabbit in the headlights of a car. See if you can identify protective figures from your life such as your parents, grandparents, pets or even made-up characters like superheroes.

Wise figures

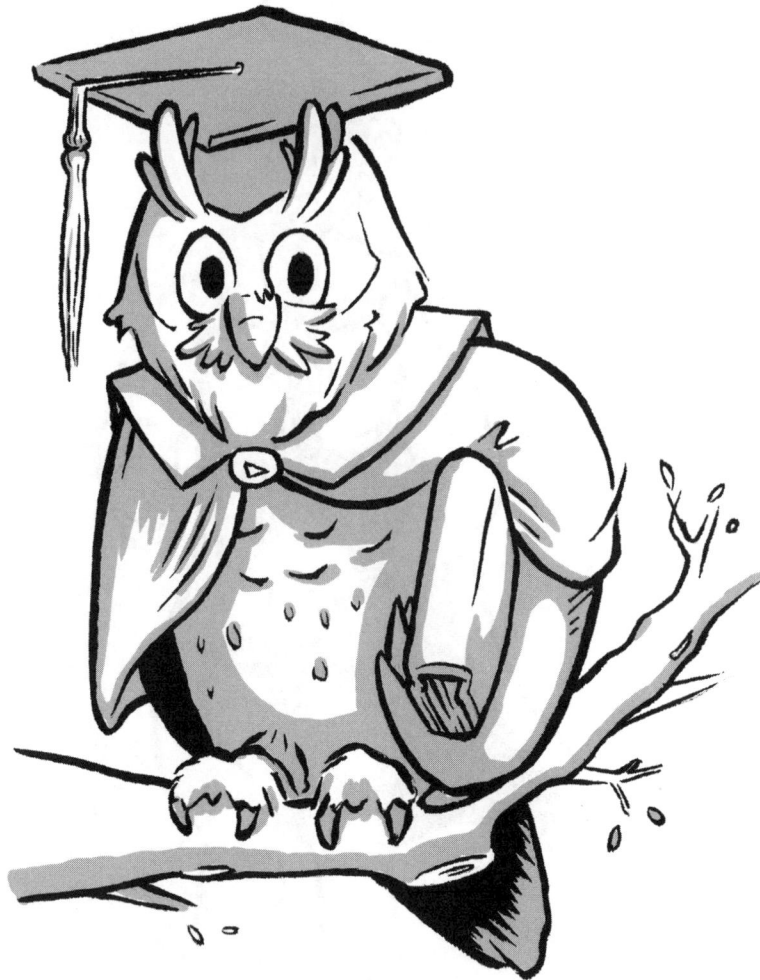

When people feel emotional or upset, it is difficult to think straight and make good decisions. Scientists have found that when we are stressed our 'thinking brain' switches off and our 'emotional brain' takes over, causing people to feel out of control and make poor choices. It is useful to call on a wise or clever person or character from your life to help out. Again, this can be someone from real life, a famous person such as Albert Einstein or even a fantasy figure, like a wizard, fairy or dragon, from your favourite film or book.

Peaceful place

Another useful resource is to imagine yourself in a peaceful, relaxing place. Everyone is different, so your imaginary places will be different also. For example, Katie imagines being on the beach on holiday with the sun shining. However, Amir likes to imagine himself playing on his Xbox. This can be a memory of somewhere special you have been in the past or it can be completely made up. Jack likes to imagine himself in Sweetie Land, while Lauren feels peaceful cuddling her pet cat Felix. In the box below, draw a picture of your own peaceful place.

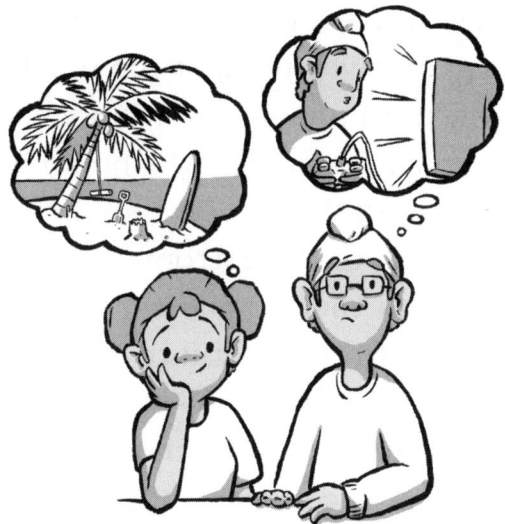

What sounds can you hear?	
Are there any smells?	
What is the weather like?	
Write a word that best describes how you feel in your picture (happy, peaceful, cool, etc.).	

Practising taking yourself to this peaceful place can help you calm down and relax when you are feeling nervous or stressed or are getting worked up.

Cool containers

Sometimes upset or scary feelings can seem too big, overwhelming or too much to bear. It can be useful to imagine putting your feelings inside a magical container which can be kept in a secret place. Perhaps you can imagine it has been dropped to the bottom of the sea or that it has a big lock that no one can open except you. Some people find it useful to actually purchase a special book or box in which to keep their feelings. Perhaps you will keep them safe until such times as you are ready to look at them again, or you can find a safe person to share them with. This can be helpful if you have upsetting feelings that come up during the week, especially if you are working together through this book with an adult helper who you don't see every day.

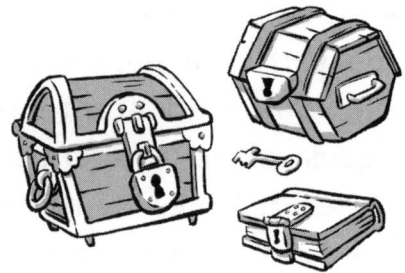

In the box below draw your own Cool Container or secret book cover. Perhaps you can also list some of the things you would put in your book or container. If the feelings or memories you want to put in the container are a secret or just too difficult to think about, you may prefer to make up a secret code or drawing to represent them. For example, 007 could represent a time you were bullied, or you could draw a circle shape to represent angry feelings.

Super special helper

Imagine that you have a special helper. This can be someone who is amazing and fantastic and can cope with anything. Perhaps they are a superhero, a fairy, a magician or a ninja. They can be real or made up. This person can be very powerful, wise or even magical. It's up to you.

Because your super special helper is able to achieve anything, they have great powers, but they are always kind and never hurt anyone. Although they can't always make bad things disappear, they can help you cope. Draw your super special helper in the box below. Perhaps your super special helper will fly like Superman or do magic like a wizard or fairy. Perhaps they are strong like Stone Man or perfectly loving like a puppy or pet unicorn.

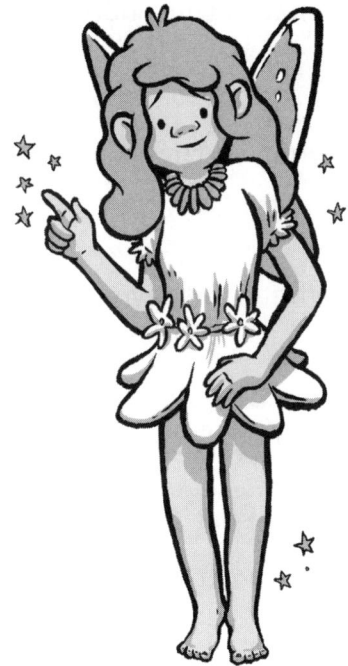

In the table below tell me in as much detail as you can about your super special helper (SSH).

What is their name?
What do they look like?
What are they wearing? (Include colours, etc.)
How do they sound?
Are they carrying or holding anything?
What super powers do they have (fly, do magic, invisible, etc.)?
How do you call your SSH to help you (whisper a magic word, rub a secret badge, spin round, etc.)?
What do they say or do to you when they come to make you feel better about yourself and the situation? (Do they comfort or cuddle you/say they will protect or help you, etc.?)
Do they give you anything to help you cope (magic stone or shield, calming powder, sleepy dust, etc.)?
What happens to your SSH when they have helped you? Where do they go?

It may be useful to think of a time in the past or the future when you have needed or may need your SSH. Write or draw a picture to show how your super special helper could help you cope in the past or will help you in the future.

Home activity 2: Resource figures

See if you can use the resources you have learned about in this session. Write in the table below any examples of times you may have used the following resources. For example, 'I used my protective figure to help me overcome some mean boys in school' or 'I felt sad during break so I went to my calm place and called my super special helper.'

Nurture or comfort figure	
Protective figure	
Wise figure	
Calm place	
Cool container	
Super special helper	

SESSION 3: IDENTIFY DIFFERENT FEELINGS

Aims and objectives

- Learn about different feelings.

- Notice how others may be feeling by looking at their faces and body language.

- Learn how feelings change all the time throughout each day.

- Begin seeing a connection between the way we feel and what we think.

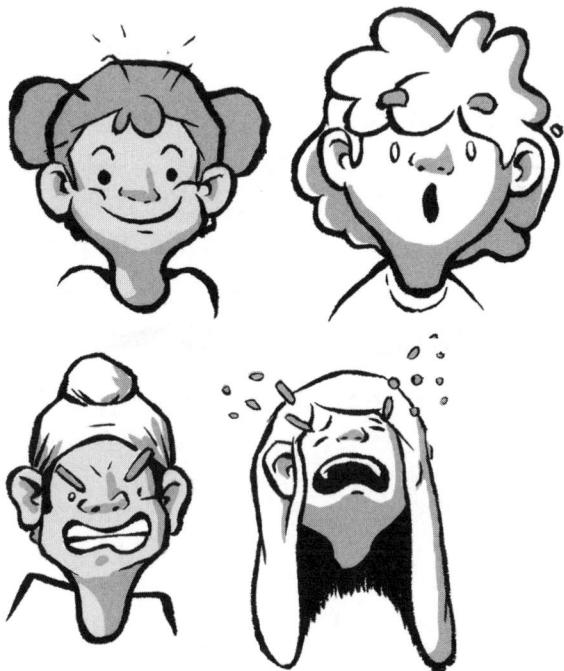

Materials

Pencils, drawing paper, feelings dice (cube or square box with different feelings – happy, sad, worried, etc. – stuck to each side).

Agenda and tips for running the session

Exercises in bold in the left-hand column should be included in both long and short sessions. Many fun activities and games are included as optional. Despite sometimes being short of time it is important not to cut all the 'fun' out of the programme or you will lose the children's enthusiasm.

Short session

EXERCISE	COMMENT
Feedback	Welcome the children and share agenda for session with the group. Obtain brief feedback from the children about their week. Perhaps one positive and one thing that has not gone so well. This feedback needs to be very brief or it can quickly consume the majority of the session. One piece of information from each child is recommended. If children provide upsetting or concerning feedback at this time empathy should be given, and one-to-one time to discuss the issue in detail is recommended following the session.
Review Home activity 2	Children can briefly feed back to the group times in the week when they used resources on their Home activity sheet. They can also share outcomes and how this was useful. It may be helpful for group facilitators to collect completed worksheets to explore in more detail following the session.
Feelings frenzy	Fun game to help children identify different feelings. A feelings dice is required.
What 'r' feelings?	Some children enjoy reading and can be made to feel more involved. However, this can slow the session down.
Name that feeling	Children are invited to share with the group and compare their answers with other group members.
Different feelings	This exercise aims to show children that people can have different feelings in the same situation. Three or four children from the group are asked to share the feelings they have identified. Group facilitators encourage the children to identify connections between their feelings and actions. For example, Jack circled that he felt scared when he saw the spider and that he would scream. Alternatively, Lauren felt excited and would pick the spider up.

Act how you feel game	As in Session 1, some children may feel self-conscious and the activity can be adapted if necessary. For example, children may act with a partner but not in front of the group.
Making cool connections	In this exercise, the children are further encouraged to make connections between how they feel and what they do. There may only be time for the children to complete one example and to share with the group if they wish. Children are encouraged to draw 'stick people' rather than complex figures to save time.
Home activity 3a: How do you feel?	This activity continues to help children make connections between their feelings and actions. It also creates an awareness of problem areas in their lives and begins to provide a range of words to describe their feelings.
Home activity 3b: Activity and feelings record	This type of activity record is frequently seen in the CBT literature. It can have many functions with regard to therapy. For the purpose of this programme, the activity record is aimed at increasing awareness of activities and the effect that these activities have on children's mood and actions. Depressed or anxious children often think that they feel like this all the time. Recording feelings in this way can be a useful way of testing this out. Children can be encouraged to do more of the activities that make them feel good and use problem-solving techniques (see Session 9) to cope better with activities that make them feel low or anxious.

Long session

More time can be spent over feedback and in the 'Act how you feel game'. Children can also be shown online clips or pictures and asked to guess the feelings of different characters. Children can be asked to discuss the characters' body language and how this can provide us with visual information about how people are feeling. Role plays are also a useful way both to portray feelings and to gain insight into the feelings of others.

Notes

All the children can be encouraged to feed back on every exercise. The session could also include online clips or picture cards showing different feelings. These could be used as an alternative to the 'Feelings frenzy' activity. Children have to identify different feelings and suggest what this tells them from what they can hear/see that the person in the picture is experiencing.

Feelings frenzy

- All children sit in a circle facing each other.

- One child volunteers to start in the middle. He/she throws the feelings dice. Depending what feeling the dice lands on, he/she must name a time, place or situation which goes with that feeling. For example: scared = when I saw a spider; excited = going to the fairground.

- After naming a place or situation, the child in the centre of the circle shouts 'feelings frenzy'.

- Any children who would share that feeling in the given situation change seats. Anyone who would not share the feeling stands on their chair.

- The person left without a chair is next to throw the feelings dice.

Example: Lauren is in the middle of the circle. She throws the feelings dice which lands on a happy face. She informs the group that she is happy when she is at home. Jack does not feel happy at home, so he stands on his chair. Amir and Katie do feel happy at home, so they rush to change places. Lauren beats Amir to Katie's seat, leaving Amir in the middle to start the game again.

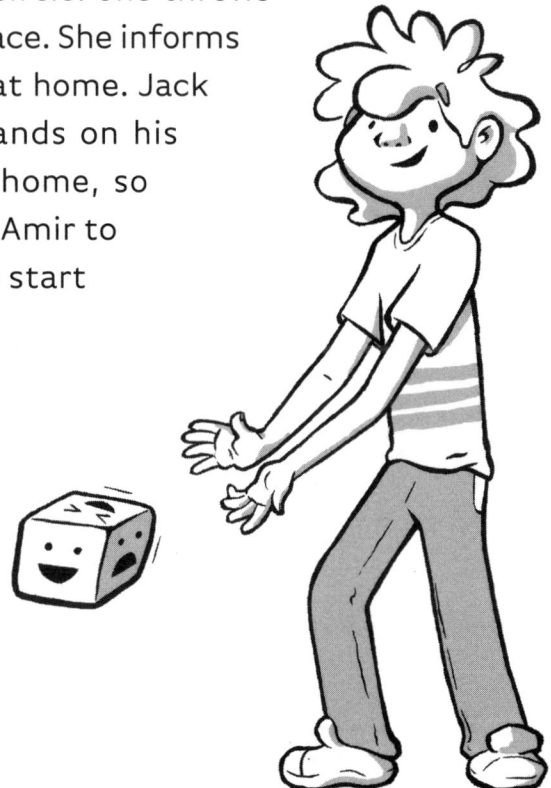

What 'r' feelings?

We all experience different feelings. They are what we feel inside about people, places or situations, for example happy, sad, angry or afraid. Becoming able to identify and name different feelings is the first important step to making cool connections about yourself and other people.

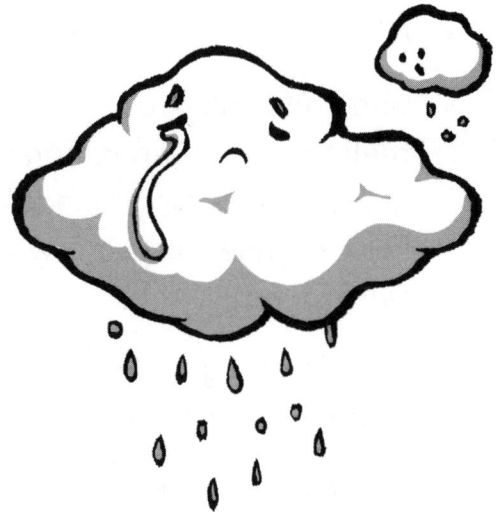

Share an example of a feeling with the rest of the group. Notice how many different feelings there are.

Feelings can change from minute to minute and day to day depending on your situation. For example, if you are running in a race you may feel happy or excited, yet if by accident you fall over and hurt yourself, your feelings may change and you become upset or angry.

In the box below, describe a time when you noticed your feelings change from one feeling to another very suddenly.

Some people think that feelings are good or bad but that is not true. They are just feelings, and feelings are neither good nor bad. It is OK to feel angry, upset or worried. It is also OK to tell others how you feel, but it is not OK to hurt other people or break things.

Sometimes people can have more than one different type of feeling at the same time.

For example:

- Jack loved his younger sister because she was good fun, but he also hated her for breaking his favourite game.

- Lauren felt really excited about going on a fairground ride but she also felt a bit nervous too.

- The man was happy and sad about a pet who died (happy his pet was no longer in pain but sad that his pet is no longer with him).

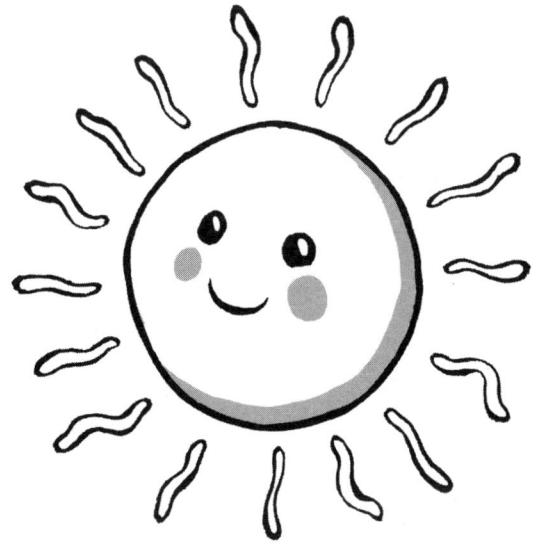

Can you share with the group a time that you had more than one feeling at the same time?

Name that feeling

You can sometimes tell how other people are feeling by looking at their faces. From the list at the bottom of the page, make cool connections by linking the face with the feeling. There are no right or wrong answers. It's up to you.

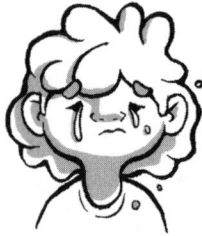

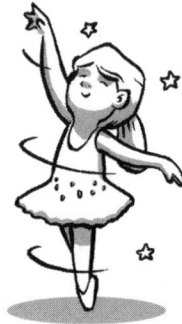

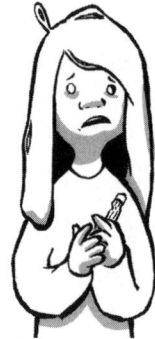

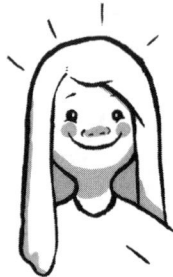

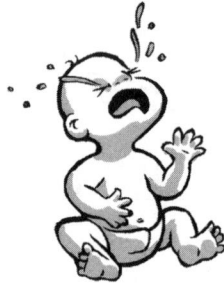

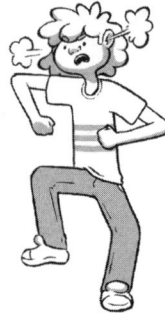

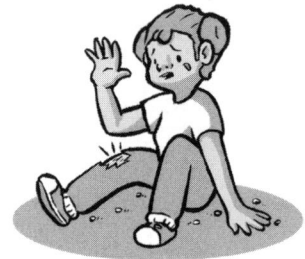

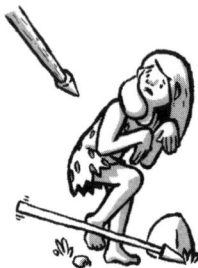

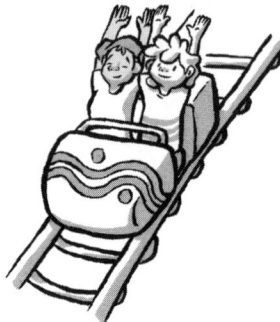

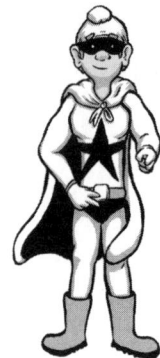

Happy	Excited	Frustrated	Upset	Tearful
Angry	Scared	Sad	Joyful	Powerful

Different feelings

Before you came to this group today, how were you feeling?

Excited	Nervous	Bored	Frustrated
Angry	Upset	Apprehensive	Disappointed
Overjoyed	Sad	Terrified	Relaxed

How would you feel if you saw a giant spider climbing up your chair?

Excited	Nervous	Bored	Frustrated
Angry	Upset	Apprehensive	Disappointed
Overjoyed	Sad	Terrified	Relaxed

How would you feel if a kind teacher gave you all some liquorice sweets?

Excited	Nervous	Bored	Frustrated
Angry	Upset	Apprehensive	Disappointed
Overjoyed	Sad	Terrified	Relaxed

Feed back your answers to the rest of the group.

What did you notice?

Did other children answer the same as you? What does this say about feelings?

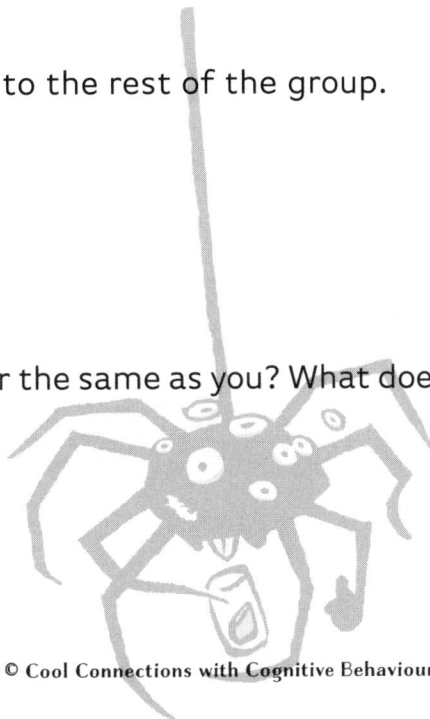

Act how you feel game

- Find a partner from within the group.

- Act or draw a situation where someone has a strong feeling. This can be real or made up (e.g. being bullied = anger; a shark attack = fear).

- Act or draw your scene and let the other group members guess what is happening. The other group members can try and identify which feelings you and your partner are demonstrating.

Briefly describe the scene you drew or acted in the box below. Which feelings were you demonstrating?

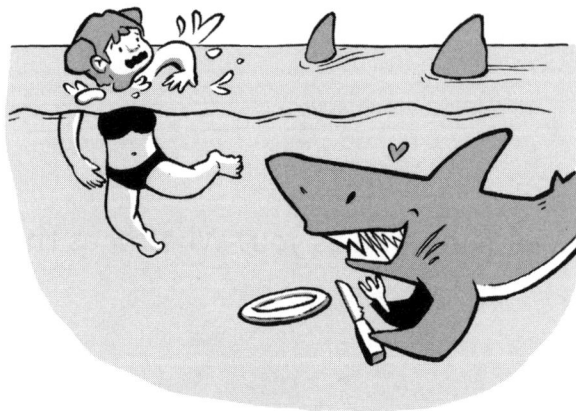

Making cool connections

Write something which makes you feel *happy*.

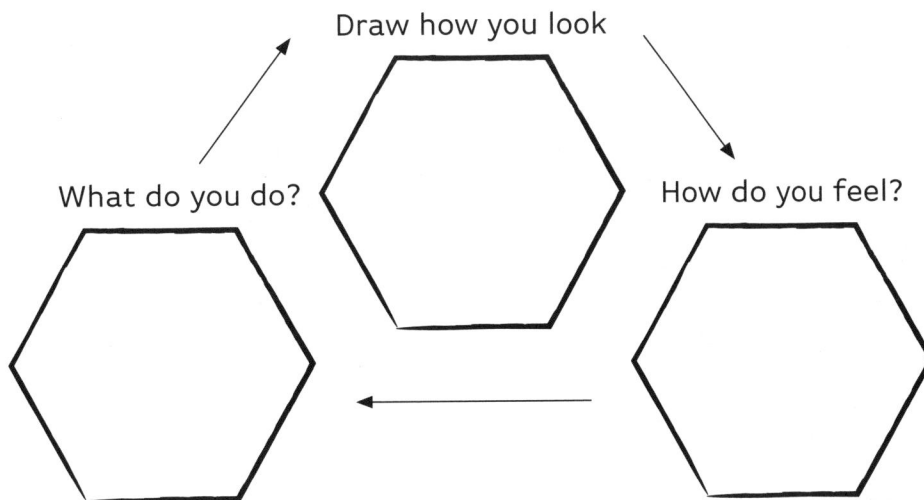

Draw how you look

What do you do?

How do you feel?

Write something which makes you feel *worried* or *scared*.

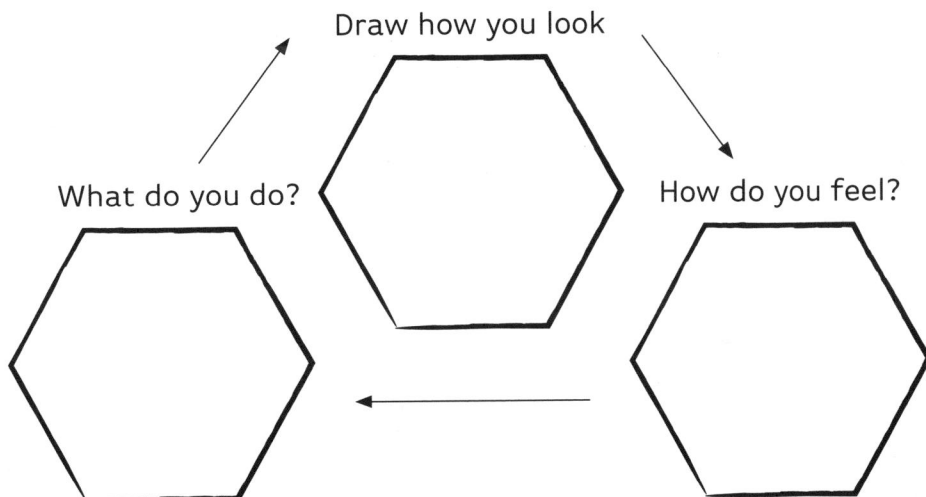

Draw how you look

What do you do?

How do you feel?

Write something which makes you feel *angry* or *cross*.

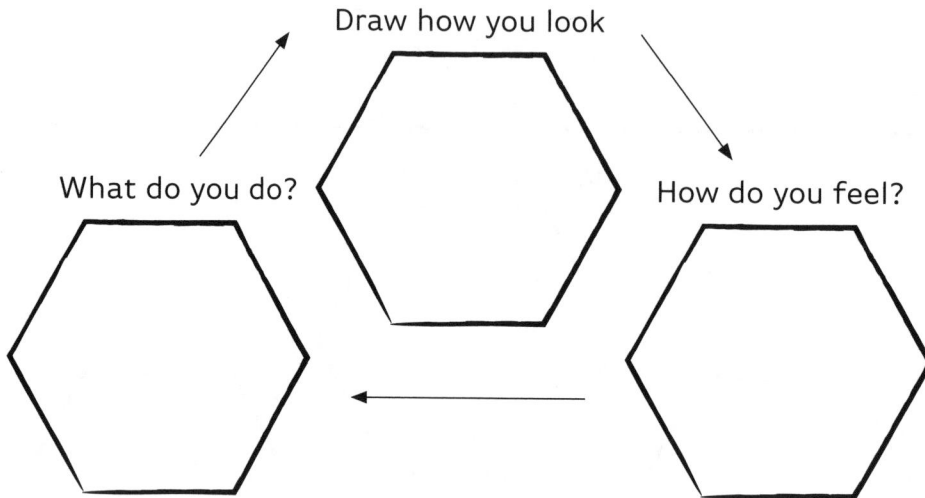

Draw how you look

What do you do?

How do you feel?

Write something which makes you feel *sad* or *down*.

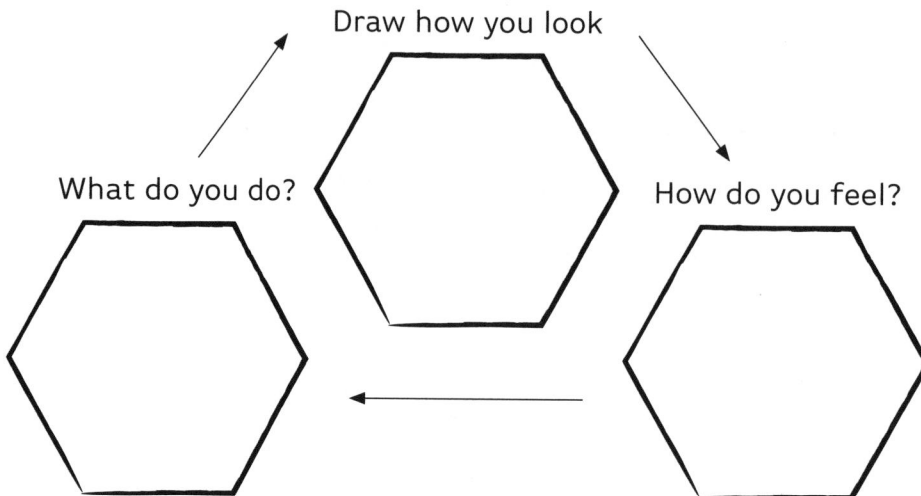

Draw how you look

What do you do?

How do you feel?

Home activity 3a: How do you feel?

Link the feelings with the situations below:

At school	In bed at night	With my friends

While out in town	Sharing my feelings	With my mum or dad

Happy	Sad	Bored
Relaxed	Angry	Frightened
Frustrated	Upset	Excited
Lonely	Guilty	Confused

Home activity 3b: Activity and feelings record

- Write the important things you have done this week in the boxes below (e.g. watching TV, maths, football, etc.).

- Write your feelings next to the activities (e.g. happy, sad, worried, etc.).

- Give your feeling a score out of 10 depending on the strength of feeling: 1 = not much, 10 = very strong.

- If you find room you could also draw what your face looked like at the time.

	MONDAY	TUESDAY	WEDNESDAY	THURSDAY	FRIDAY	SATURDAY	SUNDAY
MORNING							
LUNCH							
AFTERNOON							
EVENING							

SESSION 4: BODY SIGNALS AND BIOLOGY

Aims and objectives

- Enable the group to become aware of the physical changes in their bodies.

- Learn the connection between body signals and the way we think, feel and behave.

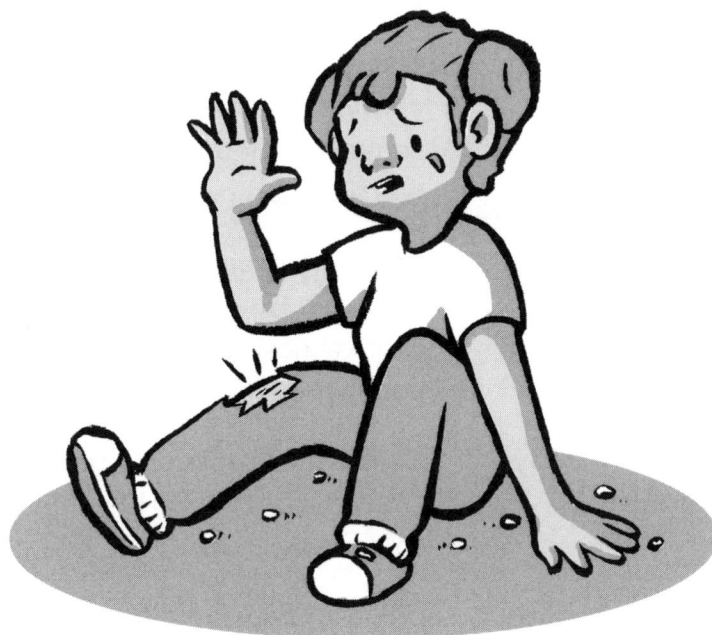

Materials

Chairs, pencils.

Agenda and tips for running the session

Exercises in bold in the left-hand column should be included in both long and short sessions. Other exercises are optional and can be included in groups where there is more time. Many fun activities and games are included as optional. Despite sometimes being short of time it is important not to cut all the 'fun' out of the programme or you will lose the children's enthusiasm.

Short session

EXERCISE	COMMENT
Feedback	Welcome the children and share agenda for session with the group. Obtain brief feedback from the children's week.
Review Home activities 3a and 3b	Children can briefly show their work. Questions may be asked about the previous week's homework. Facilitators collect home activities to explore in more detail after the session and return the following week or at the end of the programme.
Tense and floppy game	The aim is to increase children's awareness of the physical changes in their bodies and notice the difference between tense and floppy muscles. This can also be linked with worried, sad or angry feelings.
Why body signals?	Some children enjoy reading and can be made to feel more involved. However, this can slow the session down. Briefly discuss how an awareness of your body signals can prevent you losing control and help you make better choices.
Types of body signals	Children are asked to report if they have ever experienced these sensations. This helps normalise the sensations related to anxiety.
Your own body signals	Children can show their drawings and share one or two body signals that they experience with the group. It can be important for children to notice how everyone is different and that is OK. Names given for body signals can be completely made up so long as they make sense to the individual child. For example, the 'fuzzy wuzzy' feeling in my head or the 'wham bam whizzy' feeling in my tummy.
	Labelling body sensations is far more important than the quality of the drawings. 'Stick men' are fine.
What did your body do?	This exercise helps children become aware of and name their (sometimes uncomfortable) physical sensations related to their feelings. Children are encouraged to feed back one or two sensations they have identified. Many children may not be aware that other children experience similar sensations when stressed. This can be shared with the group.

Personal alarms	This helps children see that body signals associated with anxiety are intended to help us cope. They have a useful function. It may be useful for children to see that the body signals or physical sensations are exactly the same regardless of whether they are worried something bad will happen or if the bad thing actually takes place (the fear of something is sometimes more scary than the reality).
Stay cool and take it easy	This relaxation exercise is aimed at helping children become aware of physical sensations and changes within their body. If you wish, you can read from the text word for word. Alternatively, shorten or change the text to suit your group and timeframe.

Or

Experiment 4.1	It is important to check that children do not suffer with medical conditions (such as severe asthma) before taking part in this exercise. Some children may connect this experiment with uncomfortable experiences of PE at school or perhaps a time in the past when they felt very anxious. Some children may be reluctant to take part in this activity. They can be invited to watch.
Experiment 4.2	Children should be encouraged to describe the differences between the two experiments. The aim is not necessarily to encourage children to use the strategies in Experiments 4.1 and 4.2 to calm themselves down when anxious (although both may reduce symptoms in the short term) but merely to create an awareness of body sensations and to normalise these experiences.
Home activity 4: Body watching	Children are encouraged to observe others' body signals as a home activity. The aim of this activity is to further increase awareness and normalise (sometimes uncomfortable) body sensations.

Long session

Can include 'Tense and floppy game' and 'What did your body do?' Also include both 'Stay cool and take it easy' and Experiments 4.1 and 4.2. In the short session, there is too little time for all these exercises. Even in a long session you may consider that there is a lot to cover. Time permitting, children can also be encouraged to do some fun exercises at the beginning of the session such as running on the spot or playing tag. Ask them what they notice in their bodies (heart rate increases, heavy breathing, etc.). What do they notice when looking at each other? In addition, online clips or pictures can be shown and children encouraged to guess how characters are feeling from looking at their body signals.

Notes

Experiments 4.1 and 4.2 are aimed at helping children become aware of their physiology and body signals. It may also be useful to help children explore the effects of changing their physiology on the way they feel emotionally. Children can conclude what they like about the exercises and their thoughts can be discussed openly in the group. For example, 'What was different about the two experiments?', 'What do the experiments teach us about our body signals?', 'Does this have a link with anxious feelings?' Some group facilitators running short sessions may seek advice about including 'Stay cool and take it easy' or Experiments 4.1 and 4.2. As a guide, although both exercises are intended to increase children's awareness of body signals, research suggests progressive muscle relaxation ('Stay cool and take it easy') is more useful for generalised anxiety (ongoing worries about 'everything and everyone'). However, Experiments 4.1 and 4.2 have been reported to be more fun. A greater contrast between body tension and relaxation is also observed by the children.

Tense and floppy game

The game is played like musical statues without music. The group members run around the room. When asked to 'tense' they stop running and assume a tense position. When the facilitator shouts 'floppy' the group assume a relaxed position.

List what you noticed when your body became tense	List what you noticed when your body became floppy

This game helps us:

- learn about the difference between tense and relaxed (floppy)

- become more aware of the physical changes in our bodies.

Why body signals?

Another important cool connection is learning how to identify and listen to your body signals. Our bodies are changing all the time, minute by minute throughout each day, depending on how we feel. You are probably unaware of these changes unless you experience a very strong feeling such as fear or anger.

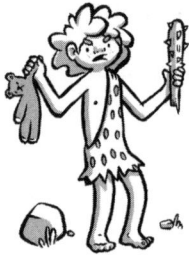

Thousands of years ago when we lived in caves, people had to fight to survive. Cavemen didn't know any other way. They may have been threatened by wild animals who wanted to eat them or maybe someone had stolen their food or taken their home.

Today we are rarely attacked by wild animals. Instead we more often feel threatened by other human beings and what they may think of us. For example, 'Am I too fat or too thin?', 'I can't do the work at school', 'Will I fail my exams?', 'What will happen if I do?' Although these fears are not life or death threats, our bodies don't always know the difference, so we react in much the same way our cavemen ancestors reacted when wild animals attacked them.

Uncomfortable feelings such as anger or fear send strong signals or messages to all parts of the body to help prepare us to fight or run away from danger. This is sometimes called the fight-or-flight response. Suddenly, hundreds of changes take place inside our bodies and we become 'pumped up' and ready for action. Our hearts pound faster, giving energy to our muscles, and we become tense and strong. Within a split second we can be ready to start a fight or run for our lives.

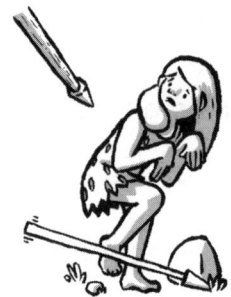

During this session we are going to become more aware of our body signals and the connections between them and our feelings. Recognising and naming body signals will help us make choices about what action to take. It may also help prevent our feelings spiralling out of control like a speeding car on the motorway without any brakes.

Unaware of body signals

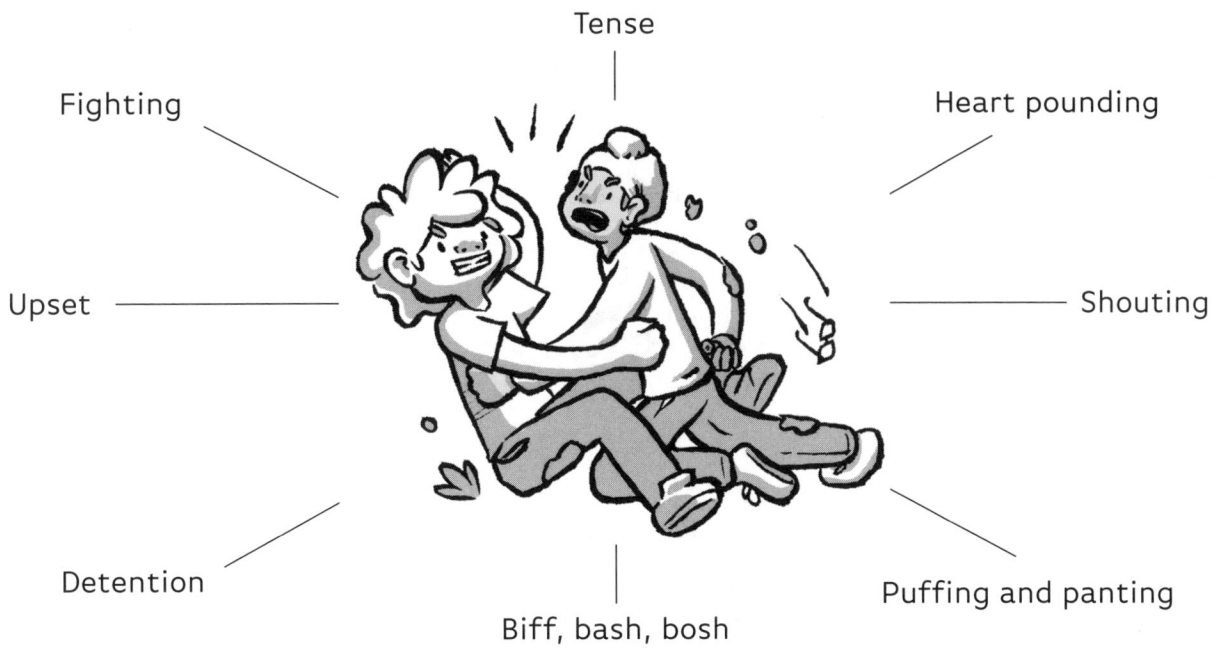

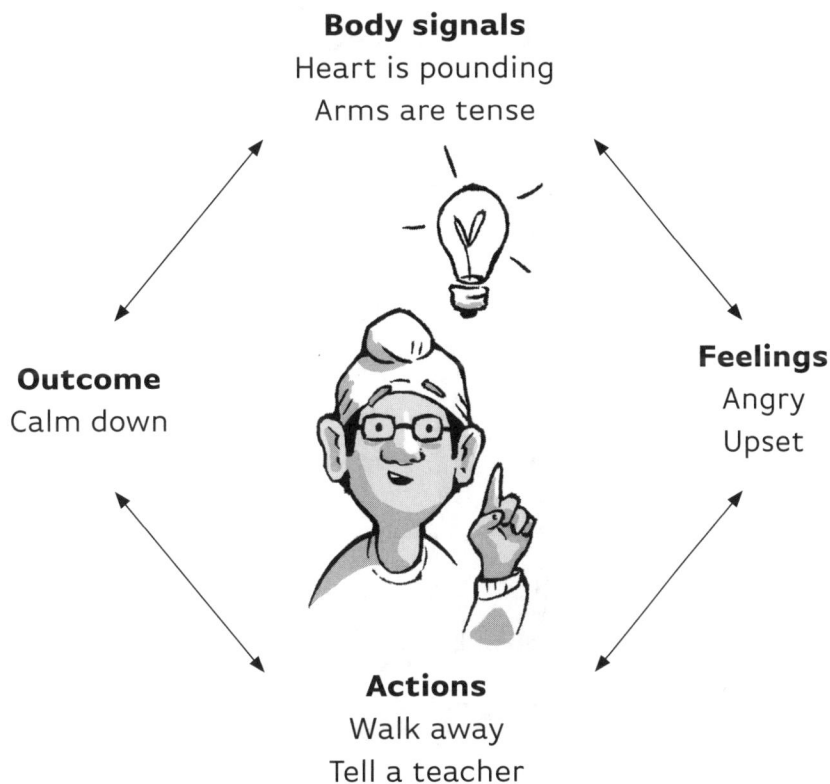

Tense

Fighting

Heart pounding

Upset

Shouting

Detention

Puffing and panting

Biff, bash, bosh

Aware of body signals

Body signals
Heart is pounding
Arms are tense

Outcome
Calm down

Feelings
Angry
Upset

Actions
Walk away
Tell a teacher

Types of body signals

It's important to learn the cool connections between your body signals when you are scared or worried.

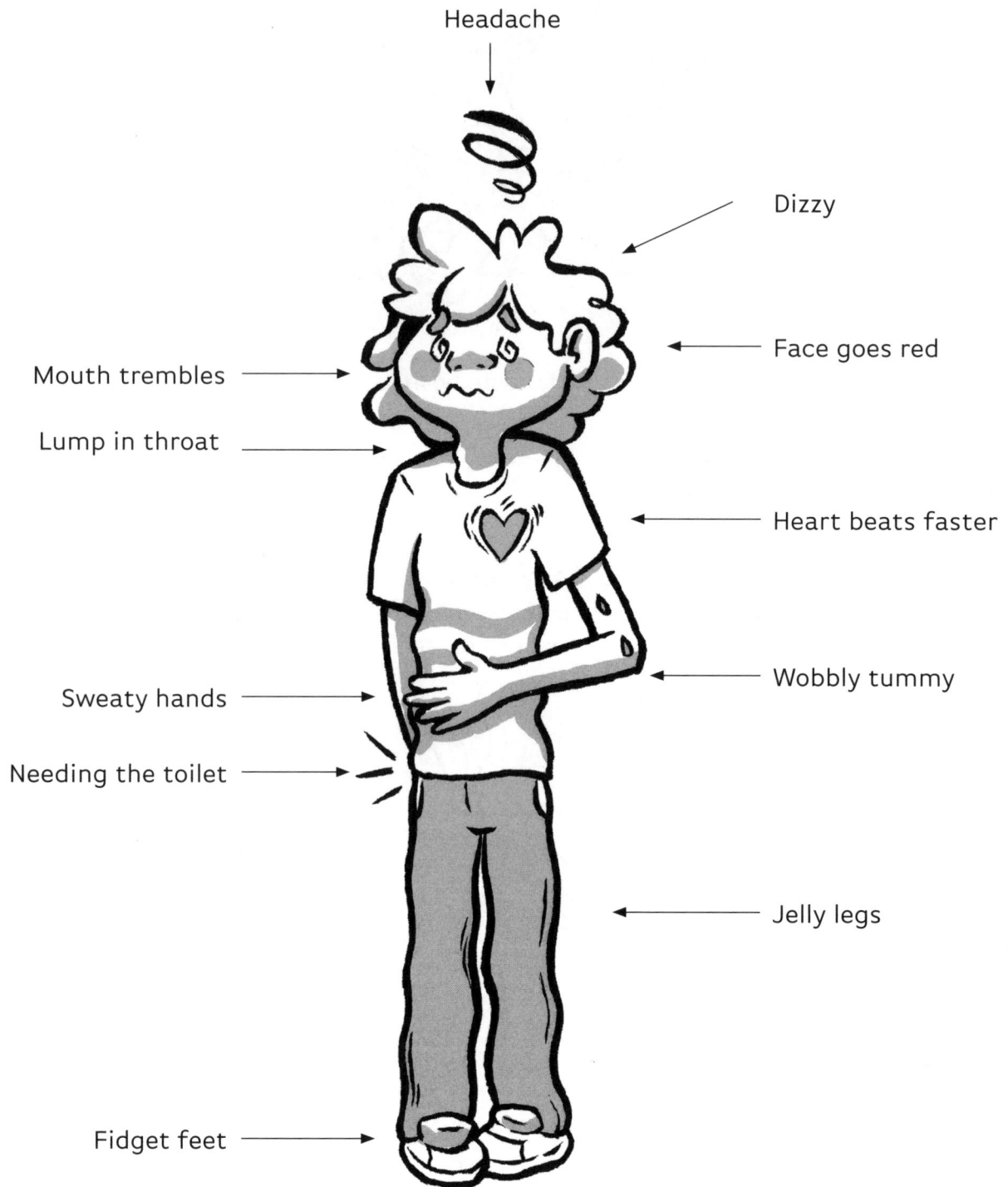

Headache

Dizzy

Face goes red

Mouth trembles

Lump in throat

Heart beats faster

Sweaty hands

Wobbly tummy

Needing the toilet

Jelly legs

Fidget feet

Your own body signals

Draw your own body in the box below showing your body signals when you are scared or worried. Everyone is different, so your signals may be different from other people in your group.

What did your body do?

Draw yourself as a stick person and show with labels what happened to your body at a time you felt the following feelings:

Excited

Angry

Frightened

Personal alarms

We all experience body signals. These signals are like a personal alarm inside us preparing our bodies for action. Our bodies quickly become pumped up and ready to fight or take flight and run away quickly. If you think back to a time when you felt upset or worried, you may have noticed your body change. Here are some of the changes and the possible reasons for them:

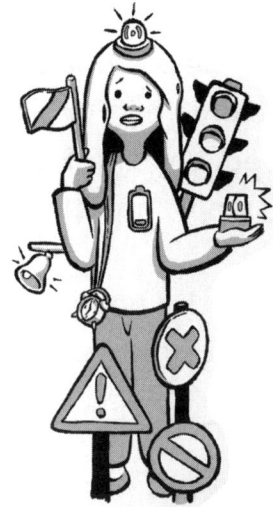

Body signals	Possible reasons
Sweating Needing the toilet	Your body needs to lose fluids so it is lighter and you can run away faster or fight better.
Breathing quickly/heavily	Your heart and lungs need more oxygen so that blood can be pumped to your muscles quickly, ready for action.
Numb or tingling hands and feet Dizziness Wobbly feelings	Blood rushes away from your hands and feet to the lungs and main muscles in your body so that you are stronger and can fight or take flight better.
Tense muscles Heart beating fast	The blood needs to be pumped round your body faster. Tense muscles make you more powerful and look more scary to an attacker.

If we did not experience body signals we would not be aware of pain or physical pleasure. We could even do our bodies some serious damage. Think, for example, what might happen if you kept walking on a broken leg or felt no pain after a serious bang on the head. Doctors would be very stuck working out what was wrong. We would not be able to tell the doctor which part of our bodies needed treatment.

The main job of body signals is to tell our brains what is happening in our bodies so that we can keep ourselves safe. Body signals themselves are always intended to be helpful. They are never bad or harmful. They are just body signals (headache, dizziness, shaking, etc.). However, the meaning we attach to these signals can often make us feel that we are in more danger than we really are. For example, you hear a noise downstairs while you are asleep in bed. You think someone is breaking in. When you go to look, you find that it is only the cat coming in through the cat flap.

List the body signals that you may have if you are lying in bed at night and you think there is a burglar downstairs in your house.

List the body signals you may have if you go downstairs and there really is a burglar walking around in your house.

What do you notice about the body signals in the above situations?

Stay cool and take it easy

Today we're going to try some exercises to help us become more aware of our body signals and the physical changes that take place when we tense and relax. Exercises like these can help you learn to relax when you are feeling uptight or get those butterfly feelings in your stomach. They're also quite clever because you can learn how to do some of them without anyone really noticing.

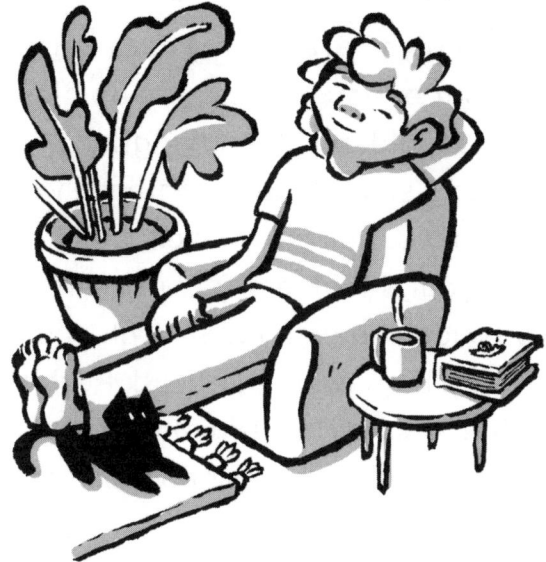

In order for you to get the best feelings from these exercises, there are some rules you must follow. First, you must do exactly what I say, even if it seems kind of silly. Second, you must pay attention to your bodies and to how your muscles feel when they are tight and when they are loose and relaxed. Third, you must practise. The more you practise, the more relaxed you can become. Before we start, get as comfortable as you can in your chair. Sit back, put both feet on the floor, and just let your arms hang loose. Now close your eyes and don't open them until I say so. Remember to follow the instructions very carefully, try hard and pay attention to your body signals.

Hands and arms

Pretend you have a whole lemon in your left hand. Now squeeze it hard. Try to squeeze all the juice out. Feel the tightness in your hand and arm as you squeeze. Now drop the lemon. Notice how your muscles feel when they are relaxed. Take another lemon and squeeze. Try to squeeze this one harder than you did the first one. That's right. Really hard. Now drop the lemon and relax. See how much better your hand and arm feel when they are relaxed. Once again, take a lemon in your left hand and squeeze all the juice out.

Don't leave a single drop. Squeeze hard. Good. Now relax and let the lemon fall from your hand. Repeat the process for the right hand and arm.

Arms and shoulders

Pretend you are a furry, lazy cat. You want to stretch. Stretch your arms out in front of you. Raise them up high over your head. Right back. Feel the pull in your shoulders. Stretch higher. Now just let your arms drop back to your side. OK, let's stretch again. Stretch your arms out in front of you. Raise them over your head. Pull them back, pull hard. Now let them drop quickly. Good. Notice how your shoulders feel more relaxed. This time let's stretch really hard. Try to touch the ceiling. Stretch your arms way out in front of you. Raise them way up high over your head. Push them way, way back. Notice the tension and pull in your arms and shoulders. Hold tight. Great. Now let them drop very quickly and feel how good it is to be relaxed.

Jaw

You have a giant jawbreaker bubble gum in your mouth. It's very hard to chew. Bite down on it. Hard! Let your neck muscles help you. Now relax. Just let your jaw hang loose. Notice how good it feels just to let your jaw drop. OK, let's tackle that jawbreaker again now. Bite down. Hard! Try to squeeze it out between your teeth. That's good. You're really tearing that gum up. Now relax again. Just let your jaw drop off your face. It feels good just to let go and not have to fight that bubble gum.

Face and nose

Here comes a really annoying fly. He has landed on your nose. Try to get him off without using your hands. That's right, wrinkle up your nose. Make as many wrinkles in your nose as you can. Scrunch your nose up real hard. Good. You've chased him away. Now you can relax your nose. Oops, here he comes back again. Right back in the middle of your nose. Wrinkle up your nose again. Shoo him off. Wrinkle it up hard. Hold it just as tight as you can. OK, he flew away. You can relax your face. Notice that when you scrunch up your nose your cheeks and your mouth and your forehead and your eyes all help you, and they get tight too. So when you relax your nose, your whole body relaxes too, and that feels good. Oh-oh. This time that old fly has come back, but this time he's on your forehead. Make lots of wrinkles. Try to catch him between all those wrinkles. Hold it tight, now. OK, you can let go. He's gone for good. Now you can just relax. Let your face go smooth, no wrinkles anywhere. Your face feels nice and smooth and relaxed.

Stomach

Imagine you can see a cute baby elephant. He's not watching where he's going. He doesn't see you lying in the grass, and he's about to step on your stomach. Don't move. You don't have time to get out of the way. Just get ready for him. Make your stomach very hard. Tighten up your stomach muscles real tight. Hold it. It looks like he is going the other way. You can relax now. Let your stomach go soft. Let it be as relaxed as you can. That feels so much better. Oops, he's coming this way again. Get ready. Tighten up your stomach. Really hard. If he steps on you when your stomach is hard, it won't hurt. Make your stomach into a rock. OK, he's moving away again. You can relax now. Kind of settle down, get comfortable, and relax. Notice the difference between a tight stomach and a relaxed one. That's how we want to feel – nice and loose and relaxed.

Legs

Now pretend that you are standing barefoot in a large dirty mud puddle. Squish your toes down deep into the mud. Try to get your feet down to the bottom of the mud puddle. You'll probably need your legs to help you push. Push down, spread your toes apart, feel the mud squish up between your toes. Now step out of the mud puddle. Relax your feet. Let your toes go loose and feel how nice it is to be relaxed. Back into the mud puddle. Squish your toes down. Let your leg muscles help push your feet down. Push your feet. Hard. Try to squeeze that puddle dry. OK. Come back out now. Relax your feet, relax your legs, relax your toes. It feels so good to be relaxed. No tenseness anywhere. You feel kind of warm and tingly.

Conclusion

Stay as relaxed as you can. Let your whole body go limp and feel all your muscles relaxed. In a few minutes, I will ask you to open your eyes, and that will be the end of this practice session. As you go through the day, remember how good it feels to be relaxed. Sometimes you have to make yourself tighter before you can be relaxed, just as we did in these exercises. Practise these exercises every day to get more and more relaxed. A good time to practise is at night after you have gone to bed and the lights are out and you won't be disturbed. It will help you get to sleep. Then, when you are really a good relaxer, you can help yourself relax at school. Just remember the elephant or the jawbreaker or the mud puddle and you can do our exercises and nobody will know. Today is a good day, and you are ready to feel very relaxed. You've worked hard and it feels good to work hard. Very slowly, now, open your eyes and wiggle your muscles around a little. Very good.

Adapted from Koeppen, A.S. (1974) 'Relaxation training for children.' *Elementary School Guidance and Counseling*, 9, 14–21.

Experiment with exercise 4a

In this exercise, we are going to experiment and make cool connections by becoming more aware of the effects of physical exercise on our bodies.

Stand up and run on the spot for between 30 seconds and one minute before completing the boxes below. What body signals and sensations are you aware of right now?

What do you notice about your heart rate and your breathing?

What do you think might happen if you kept doing this exercise?

Write about a time that you have experienced these body signals before.

Experiment with relaxation 4b

Breathe slowly and deeply, counting in 2–3 and out 2–3. Imagine you are on a sunny beach with the waves gently lapping against the sea shore. Breathe deeply for about a minute. Let your stomach rise and fall. Imagine your stomach is like the tides of the sea. As you breathe out, slowly imagine the tide coming in again like a wave.

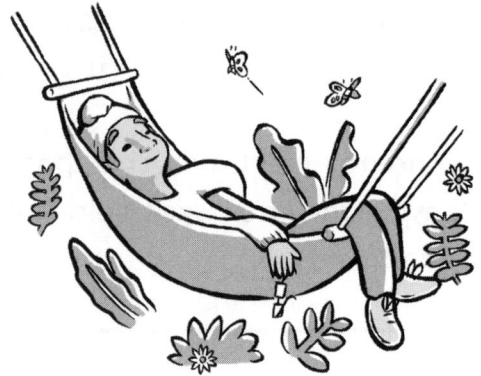

What body signals and sensations are you aware of right now?

What do you notice about your heart rate and your breathing?

What do you think might happen if you kept doing this exercise?

Write about a time that you have experienced these body signals before.

In Experiments 4.1 and 4.2 you were encouraged to become more aware of your body signals. Write anything that you noticed about the experiments in the box below. Have you learned anything that might help you next time you feel scared or worried?

Home activity 4: Body watching

Red face (blushing)	Dry mouth (lip smacking)	Sweating	Tense body (stiff)
Shaking	Heavy breathing (panting)	Choking/ retching (like being sick)	Tearful (crying/ laughing)
Screwed-up face (snarling/pain)	Clenched fists	Heart pounding (neither their pulse)	Cheeks puffed (like smiling)

Watch your friends, family and teachers this week and see if you can make cool connections by spotting all the body signals written above. Write them in the table below:

Body signal	Child = C Adult = A	What are they doing at the time?
Example: Red face	A	Shouting at a group of naughty children in school

SESSION 5: IDENTIFYING THOUGHTS

Aims and objectives

- Help identify thoughts.

- Learn the effect our thinking has on our feelings and actions.

Materials

Chairs, pencils, small tub or box for folded paper in Thought–feeling cool connections exercise.

Agenda and tips for running the session

Exercises in bold in the left-hand column should be included in both long and short sessions. Other exercises are optional and can be included in groups where there is more time. Many fun activities and games are included as optional. Despite sometimes being short of time it is important not to cut all the 'fun' out of the programme or you will lose the children's enthusiasm.

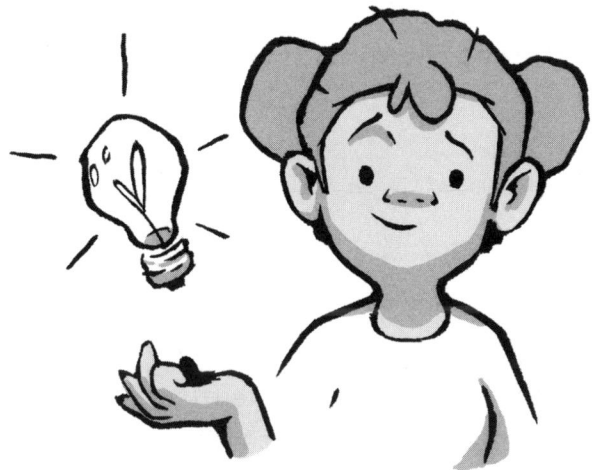

Short session

EXERCISE	COMMENT
Feedback	Welcome the children and share agenda for session with the group. Obtain brief feedback about the children's week.
Review Home activity 4	Group facilitators collect home activities from Session 4 to explore in more detail after this session and return the following week (Session 6) or at the end of the programme. Questions may be asked about the previous week's homework.
Thought whisper game	Fun way to demonstrate how thoughts can be misinterpreted. Game works best if the facilitator makes up the first short sentence to avoid confusion.
About thoughts	Some children enjoy reading and can be made to feel more involved. However, this can slow the session down.
Fill in the thought bubbles	Children begin to identify thoughts. Each child can be asked to feed back to the group one or two of the thoughts he or she has associated with the different characters on the page.
Different thoughts	Children write different thoughts about themselves than those they consider other children have about them. It is likely that the thoughts children write about other children are closely linked to thoughts/beliefs that they have about themselves. However, this cannot be taken as fact, and if appropriate this may need to be checked out with individual children. Children can be asked to feed back to the group one or two different thoughts they have identified. It is useful to help the group identify how some children think in similar ways while others think quite differently. There is no right or wrong way of thinking. Thoughts are just thoughts.

Thought–feeling cool connections

Shows the connection between thoughts and feelings. May help children begin to empathise with how others feel when children are cruel or say unkind things. It is useful to share with the group that children sometimes say unkind 'nasty' things to themselves in their own thoughts, for example 'You're stupid or weird'. Children can be questioned about how they feel inside when they think these unpleasant things about themselves. It is important that children do not write their names on the paper or personalise their unhelpful thoughts about any members of the group.

Catching thoughts example

Read the page to the children and ask what they think about these examples. Encourage the children to make connections between the way the children look, feel and think. For example, 'How do you think the children in the examples are feeling?', 'How would you feel if you had these thoughts?'

Catching thoughts

Children are encouraged to share their thoughts with the group but should not be pressurised to do so. A comment about confidentiality within the group may help children disclose more personal information.

Home activity 5: Catching thoughts

This encourages children to practise catching thoughts. Just catching thoughts can make a significant difference to the way they feel. Catching specific thoughts helps children develop awareness and begin to validate their feelings.

Long session

More time can be spent on feedback. Include 'Thought whisper game'. Children can be shown comics with examples of thought bubbles. Some self-help guides show examples of thoughts which can be shared with the children – for example, the videos associated with the *Coping Cat Series* which can be obtained from Workbook Publishing (www.workbookpublishing.com). Some films also provide excellent examples of thoughts, for example *What Women Want*, in which Mel Gibson, who acts as a sales rep, has an accident and is suddenly able to hear the thoughts of women. It can be noted how being able to hear these thoughts changes his feelings and behaviour towards the women around him. (As this film is rated age 15, consent should be obtained from parents, even if only showing a censored clip to this age group of children.) In some sessions, we have given children a cut-out of a famous character (such as Donald Duck, Superman) and played a guessing game, matching the different thoughts they may have about themselves. For example, 'What's up Doc?' and 'I love carrots' would match with Bugs Bunny, and 'I'm always on the web' or 'I am such a superhero' would match Spider-Man. This game is good fun and helps children identify with the fact that different people have different thoughts about themselves.

Notes

The exercises in this session aim to help children become aware of their thoughts. Children are informed that thoughts can also be images or 'pictures in their heads'. Some children may choose to draw their thoughts, which is fine, although not much room is provided in the text boxes.

Thought whisper game

- All children sit in a circle.

- One group member whispers a short sentence or thought to the person sitting next to them.

- This person in turn whispers what they heard to the next person, and so on round the circle.

- The last person announces what they heard.

- This game provides a fun way to show how thoughts can get misinterpreted.

- People tend to hear what they want to hear rather than what has actually been said.

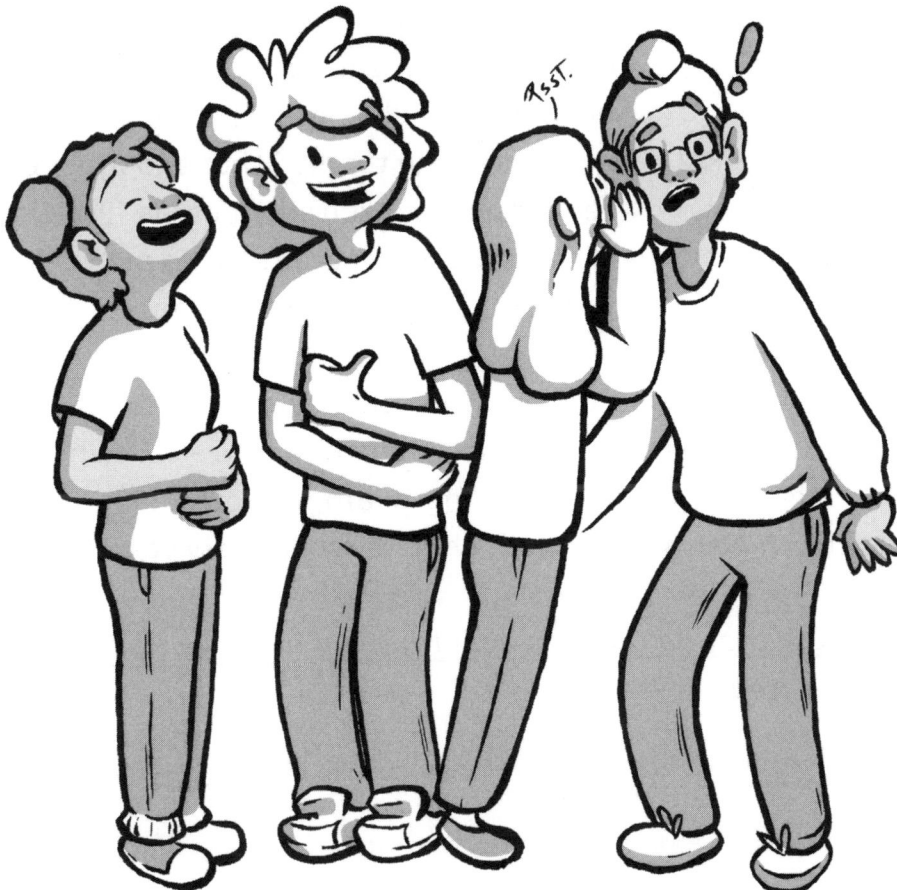

About thoughts

Everybody has thoughts, and this includes children, adults and even babies. Thoughts go on all the time in our heads. Sometimes they are like words or sentences and sometimes they are in the form of pictures, as in our dreams. We have thoughts about ourselves such as 'I'm so fantastic', thoughts about other people, for example 'I don't like her, she's horrid', and thoughts about the things around us, like 'My school is so cool' or 'The world can be a dangerous place'. Everyone is different, so everyone has different thoughts.

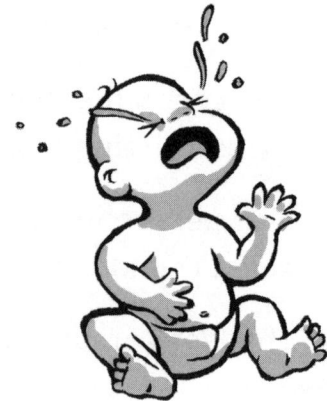

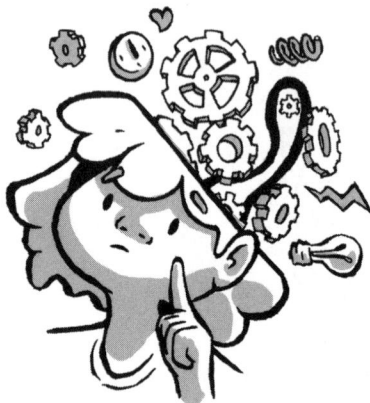

The cool connections about our thoughts are that they make a difference to how we feel and what we do. Some of the thoughts we have can make us feel angry, sad or worried. For example, 'I'm ugly, no one likes me' or 'I'm never going to get picked for the team'. Other thoughts can make us feel happy or excited, such as 'I'm the cleverest in the school, everyone loves me' or 'I'm going to the fair tonight with my mates'.

There are many people who believe that there are good and bad thoughts. However, the truth is that thoughts are just thoughts – it's what you do that makes the difference. In the following example both Jack and Katie have angry thoughts. In your view, which child is most likely to get into trouble?

Jack felt so angry that he thought about hitting his little sister but he decided to go for a run instead.

Katie thought her brother was horrid so she broke his favourite computer game.

Sometimes we are aware of our thinking, but a lot of the time our thoughts go unnoticed. By stopping and listening to your thoughts you can find out a lot about yourself and your feelings. In today's session, we will be learning more about thoughts and how to catch them so that we can find out more about ourselves.

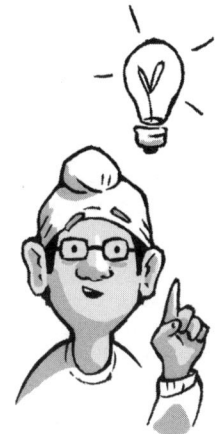

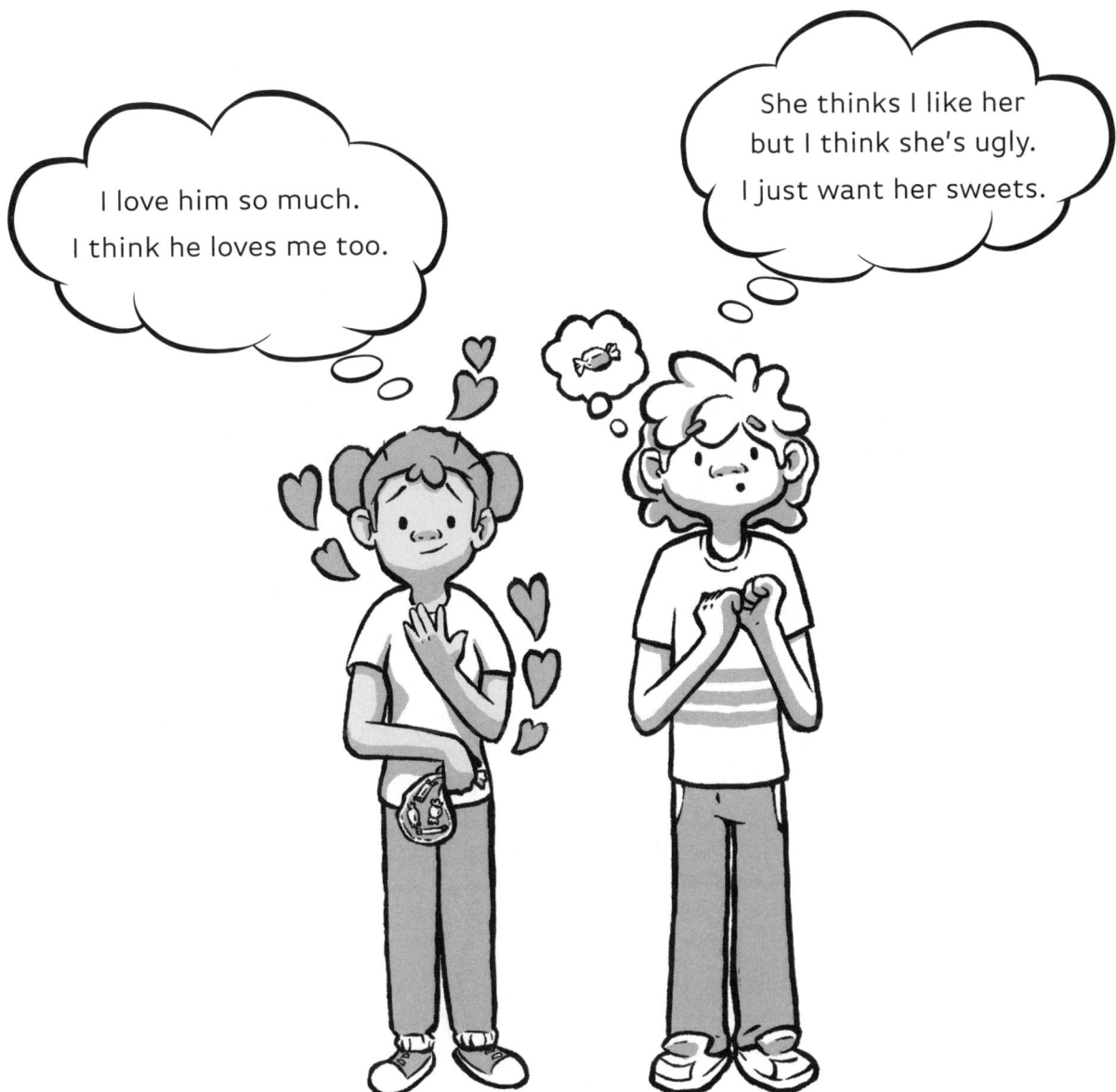

I love him so much.
I think he loves me too.

She thinks I like her but I think she's ugly.
I just want her sweets.

Fill in the thought bubbles

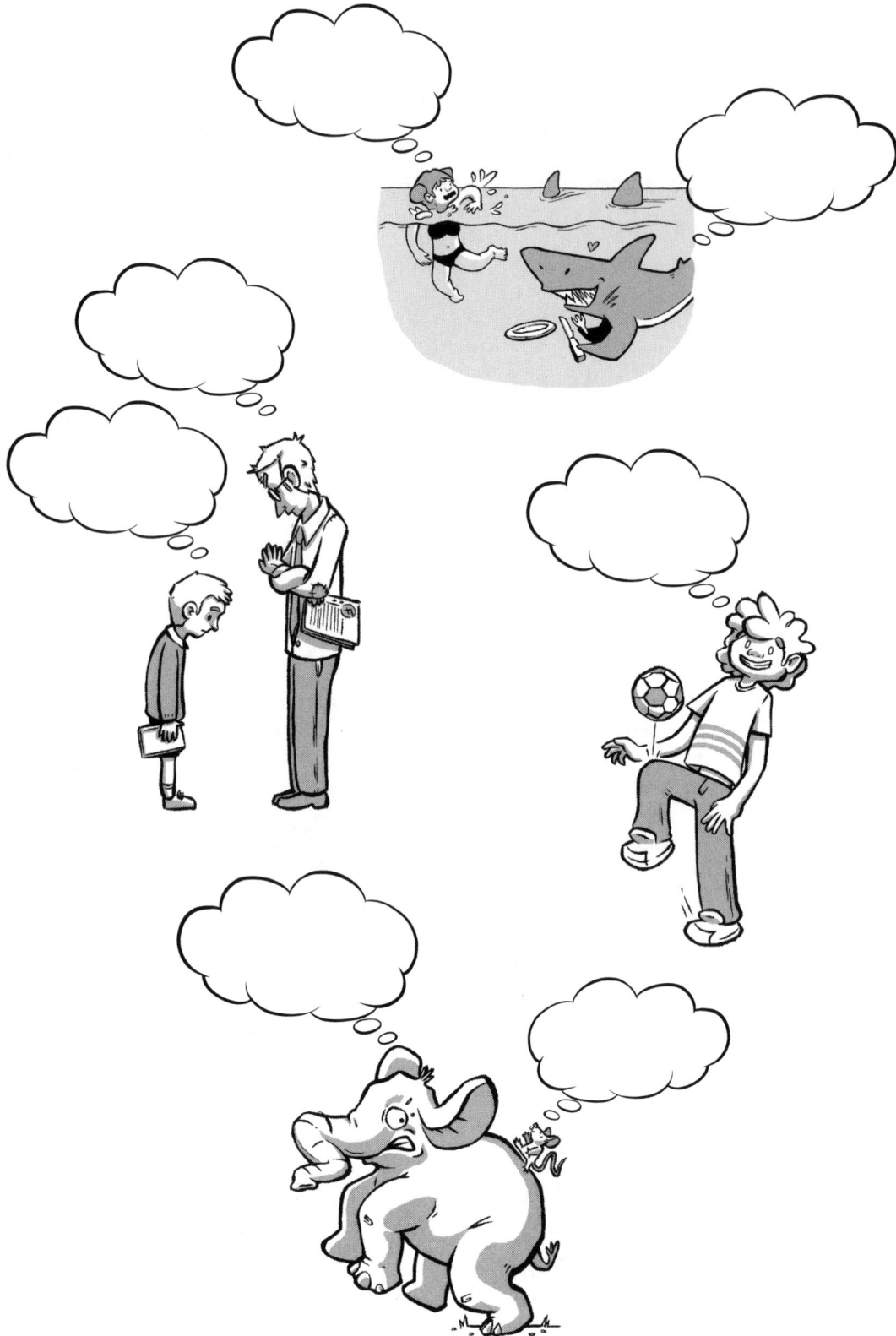

Different thoughts

All of us have different thoughts running through our minds all the time. Some of these thoughts make us feel happy inside, while others make us feel angry, sad or scared. Make cool connections by writing some of the thoughts other children may have in the different situations below:

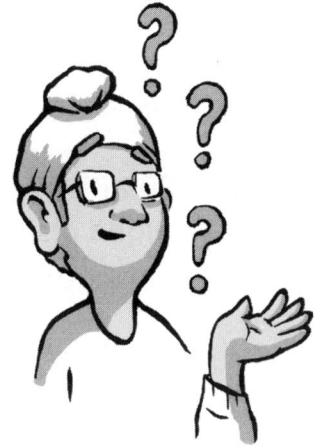

Thoughts about themselves

Happy thoughts	Sad, worried or angry thoughts

Their school

Happy thoughts	Sad, worried or angry thoughts

Their home

Happy thoughts	Sad, worried or angry thoughts

Thought-feeling cool connections

- Group members sit in a circle and each is given two small pieces of paper.

- On one piece of paper they write something that would make someone else feel good about themselves (e.g. 'I like your smile' or 'You are good fun to be with').

- On the other piece of paper they write something mean or nasty like a bully might say (e.g. 'You're horrid' or 'You are so ugly').

- All the paper messages are folded and placed anonymously in a tub or box.

- Group members take two random pieces of paper from the tub.

- Each child reads the paper messages one at a time, facing the person next to them.

- The group are asked to report how they would feel and what they would do if the statements were said to them.

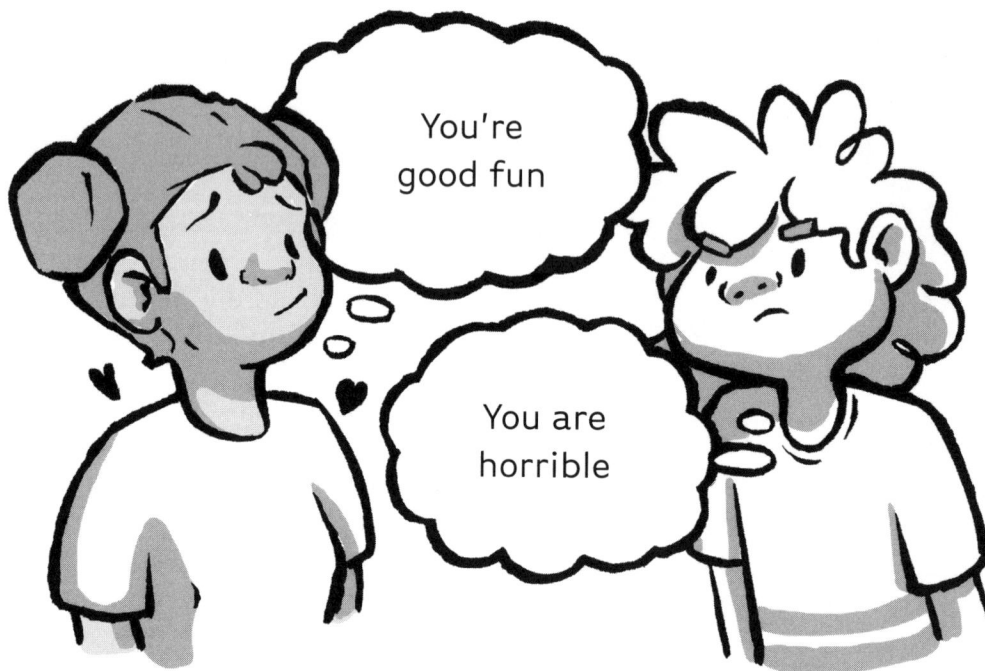

Catching thoughts example

Now that you have learned the cool connections about thoughts and feelings, look at the examples below showing Katie and Amir's thoughts and feelings in different situations. Notice how their thoughts seem to affect the way they look and feel.

What happened? Mrs Jones my English teacher told me to read out in front of the whole class.

How does my face look?

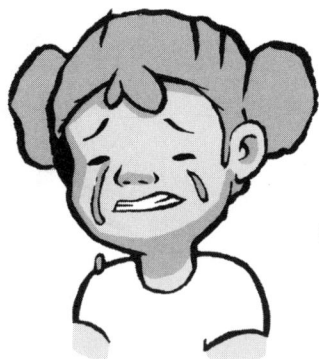

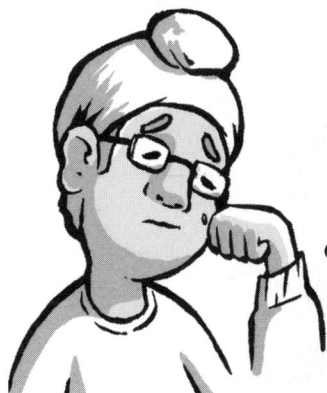

I hate Mrs Jones for making me read out loud

I will look really stupid

My face will go red and other kids will laugh

I just can't do it – arrrrrh!

What happened? Fred Bloggs pushed me in the playground and I fell over.

How does my face look?

Fred Bloggs is a nasty bully and he stinks

Why does everyone pick on me?

Everyone hates me in this school

I don't want to go to this school any more

Catching thoughts

Make cool connections between your thoughts and feelings. Next to 'What happened?', write something from the past or present that has made you feel unhappy, angry or scared. In the thoughts bubble, write or draw the thoughts you had about this. Finally, under 'How does my face look?', draw how the thoughts made you feel. If you cannot think of an example for yourself, make one up about a friend or member of your family. Good luck!

What happened? . . . .

How does my face look?

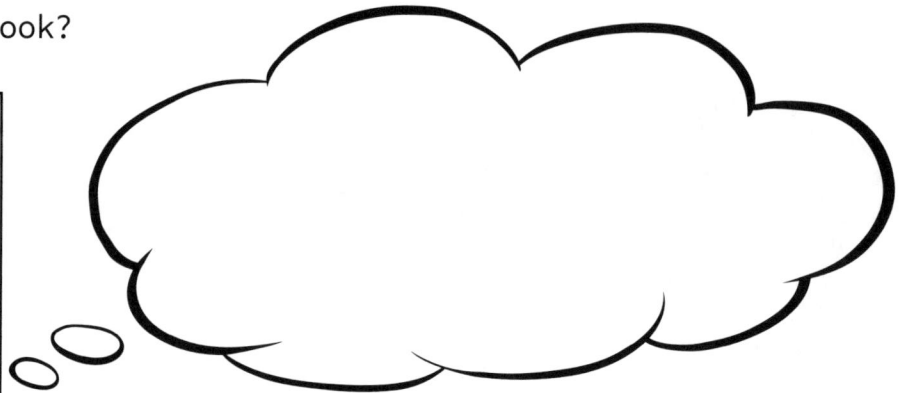

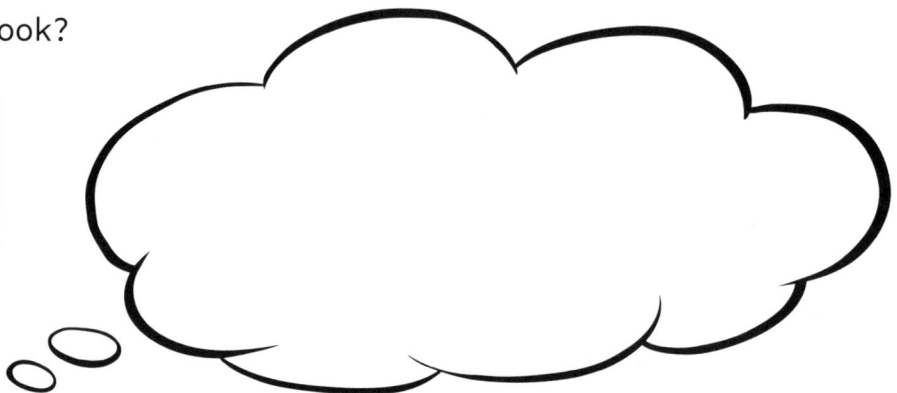

What happened? . . . .

How does my face look?

Home activity 5: Catching thoughts

In the last session, we learned about catching thoughts. Here is another chance to practise. Next to 'What happened?', write something that has happened to you that made you feel unhappy, angry or scared. In the thoughts bubble, write or draw the thoughts you had about this. Finally, under 'How does my face look?', draw what your face may have looked like at the time. If you prefer you can make up an example about a friend or a member of your family.

What happened? . . . .

How does my face look?

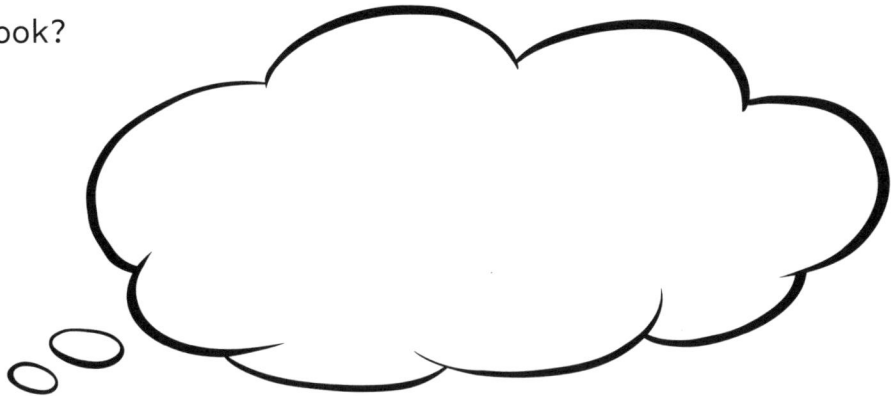

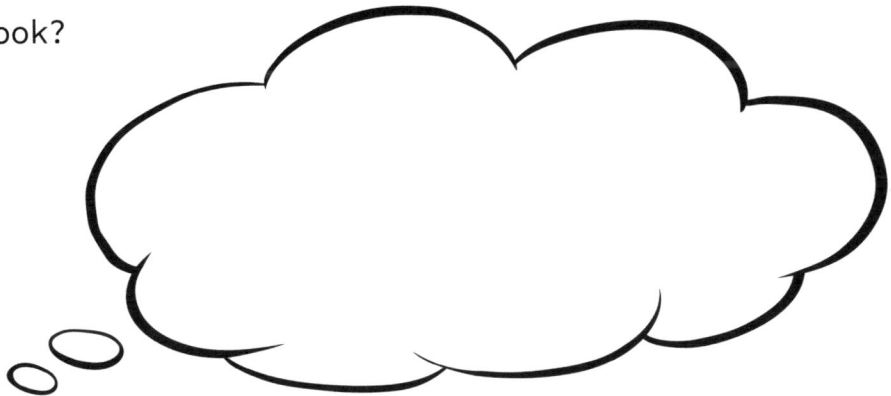

What happened? . . . .

How does my face look?

SESSION 6: THE CONNECTIONS BETWEEN THOUGHTS, FEELINGS, BODY SIGNALS AND ACTIONS

Aims and objectives

- Understand the links between thoughts, feelings, body signals and actions.

- Pull together the other sessions in the programme so far.

- See how a change in either our thinking, feelings, body signals or actions can affect the other connections.

- Notice similarities and differences between yourself and others in the group.

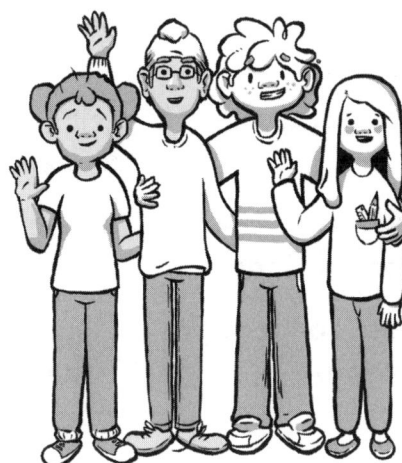

Materials

Chairs, pencils, a hoop, large paper labels with thoughts, feelings, body signals and actions written on separate pieces of paper for 'Cool connections game'.

Agenda and tips for running the session

Exercises in bold in the left-hand column should be included in both long and short sessions. Other exercises are optional and can be included in groups where there is more time. Many fun activities and games are included as optional. Despite sometimes being short of time it is important not to cut all the 'fun' out of the programme or you will lose the children's enthusiasm.

Short session

EXERCISE	COMMENT
Feedback	Welcome the children and share agenda for session with the group. Obtain brief feedback about the children's week.
Review Home activity 5	Children can briefly show work. Facilitators collect home activities to explore in more detail after the session and return the following week or at the end of the programme.
Hoops	Fun activity to help children warm up in session.
The Zog from Zen	This story is aimed at helping children begin to understand the cognitive model (links between thoughts, feelings, physical sensations and behaviour). Some children enjoy reading and can be made to feel more involved. However, this can slow the session down.
Your actions	Helps children become more self-aware by making connections between their feelings and their actions.
Different cool connections	This section can be read to the children or they can be asked to read this to themselves and then feed back to the group.
Cool connections example	Group facilitator shares an example. The group can be asked if they would have similar or different feelings, body signals, thoughts and so on to the child in the example.
My cool connections	If children cannot identify a time when they felt frightened or sad, they can either make it up or use a time when a parent or friend felt this way. There are no right or wrong answers. Children can choose to share their examples or keep them private.
Cool connections game	Use the sentences listed for the game or make up your own.
Home activity 6a: Quick quiz	This helps reinforce the cool connections learned so far. It increases facilitators' awareness of how well group members are beginning to understand the cognitive model (links between thoughts and feelings).
Home activity 6b: Cool connections	It is useful to inform children that their home activity work is kept confidential and will not be shared with the group without their consent.

Long session

More time can be spent on each exercise. Include the 'Hoops' and the 'Cool connections' games. To illustrate further the way our thoughts and feelings are linked, it can be useful to show an online clip of how someone's behaviour changes when they get new or different information. With boys, I often use a clip from the film *The Karate Kid* where the young karate student is angry with his teacher for making him paint the fence, sand the floor and wax the car. His mood and behaviour completely change when he learns that he has been learning karate techniques all along.

Notes

The exercises in this session are about gaining an awareness of thoughts, feelings, body signals and actions, and the connections between them. It is more beneficial if children are prepared to share their own material and write personal thoughts, feelings and so on in the boxes provided in the session, but this is not essential. Merely becoming aware of thoughts, feelings, body signals and actions, and the connections between them (the cognitive model), will help children develop their own emotional literacy skills. With practice, children can begin to label their own feelings and gain a better awareness of the emotional experiences of others.

Hoops

Group members stand in a circle. Each child links hands or arms with the children either side of them. One child places a hoop around themselves. The object of the exercise is to move the hoop from person to person right round the circle without using hands and breaking the connection between the children in the circle.

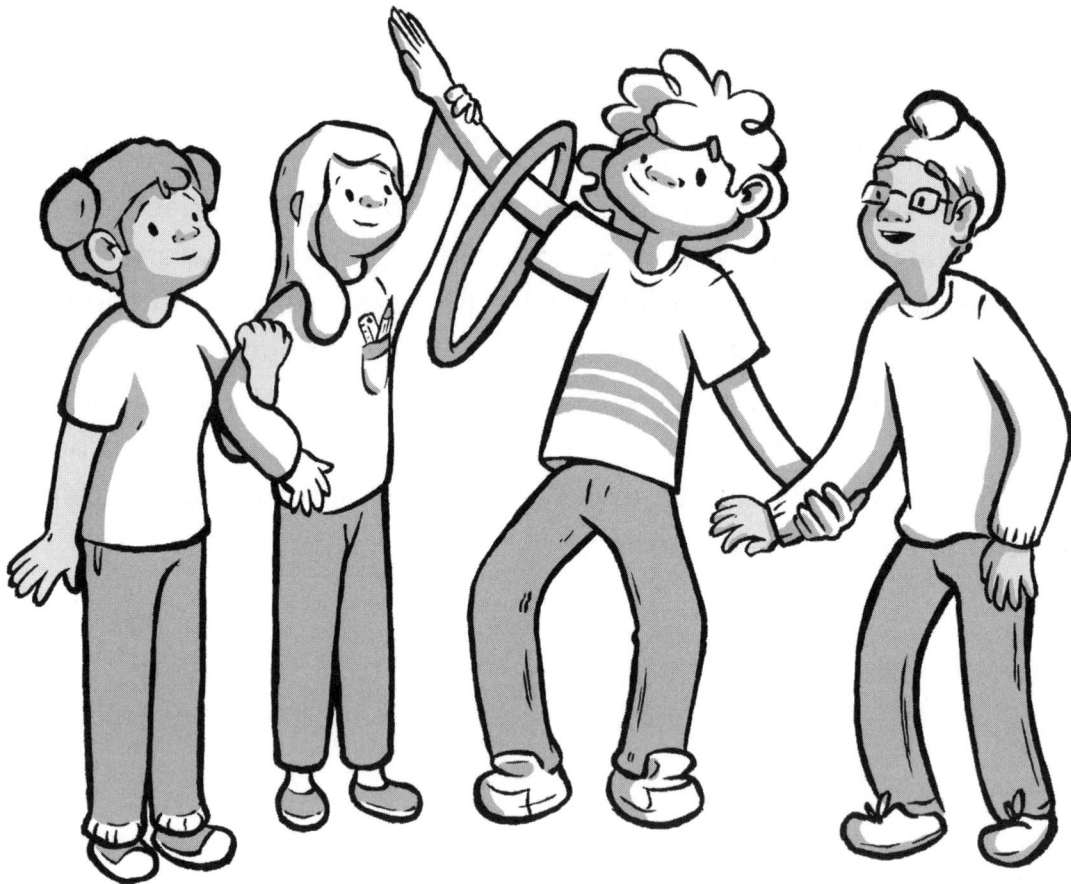

This game indicates that:

- problem-solving is easier with the help of others

- when things are connected, if one part moves it affects the other parts.

The Zog from Zen

In this session, we are going to look at the cool way that your thoughts, feelings, body signals and actions are all connected. Listen to the story below.[1]

The Zog is an alien from outer space who lives on the planet Zen. One day he woke up feeling excited because it was his birthday. The Zog's body felt tingly and he noticed a warm fuzzy feeling in his tummy. He said to himself, 'Today will be great because I'm having a party. All my Zen friends are coming. I love birthdays.' He quickly jumped out of bed, put on his Zen clothes and went off to the party at the Zen village hall.

Notice how the Zog's thoughts, feelings, body signals and actions are all connected. One part cannot move without the other.

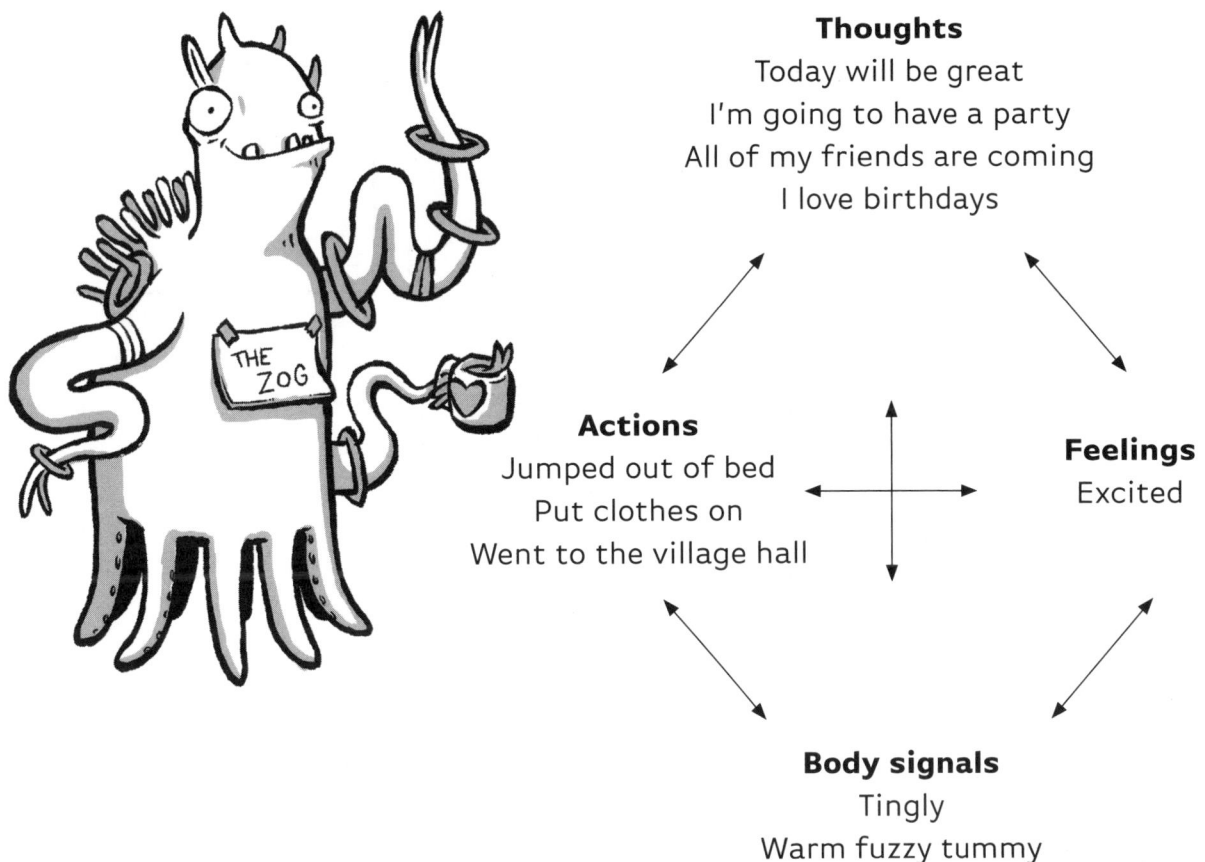

Thoughts
Today will be great
I'm going to have a party
All of my friends are coming
I love birthdays

Actions
Jumped out of bed
Put clothes on
Went to the village hall

Feelings
Excited

Body signals
Tingly
Warm fuzzy tummy

---

1   Adapted, with permission, from Friedberg, R.D. *et al.* (2001) 'Diamond Connections.' In *Therapeutic Exercises for Children: Guided Self-Discovery Using Cognitive-Behavioral Techniques* (pp.8–11). Copyright 2001 Professional Resource Exchange, Sarasota, FL.

The time came for the party to begin but no alien friends arrived. The Zog looked out of the window but he could not see any of his Zen friends arriving. As time went by the Zog began to feel sad and worried. His mouth felt dry and his throat felt as if there was a lump in it. The Zog's tummy started to turn over and over and his alien heart pounded in his chest. He thought, 'What shall I do? I've been forgotten', 'My alien friends don't like me' and 'I'm like Billy No-mates'. The Zog sat down, put his head in his hands and cried.

Can you work out what goes in each box?

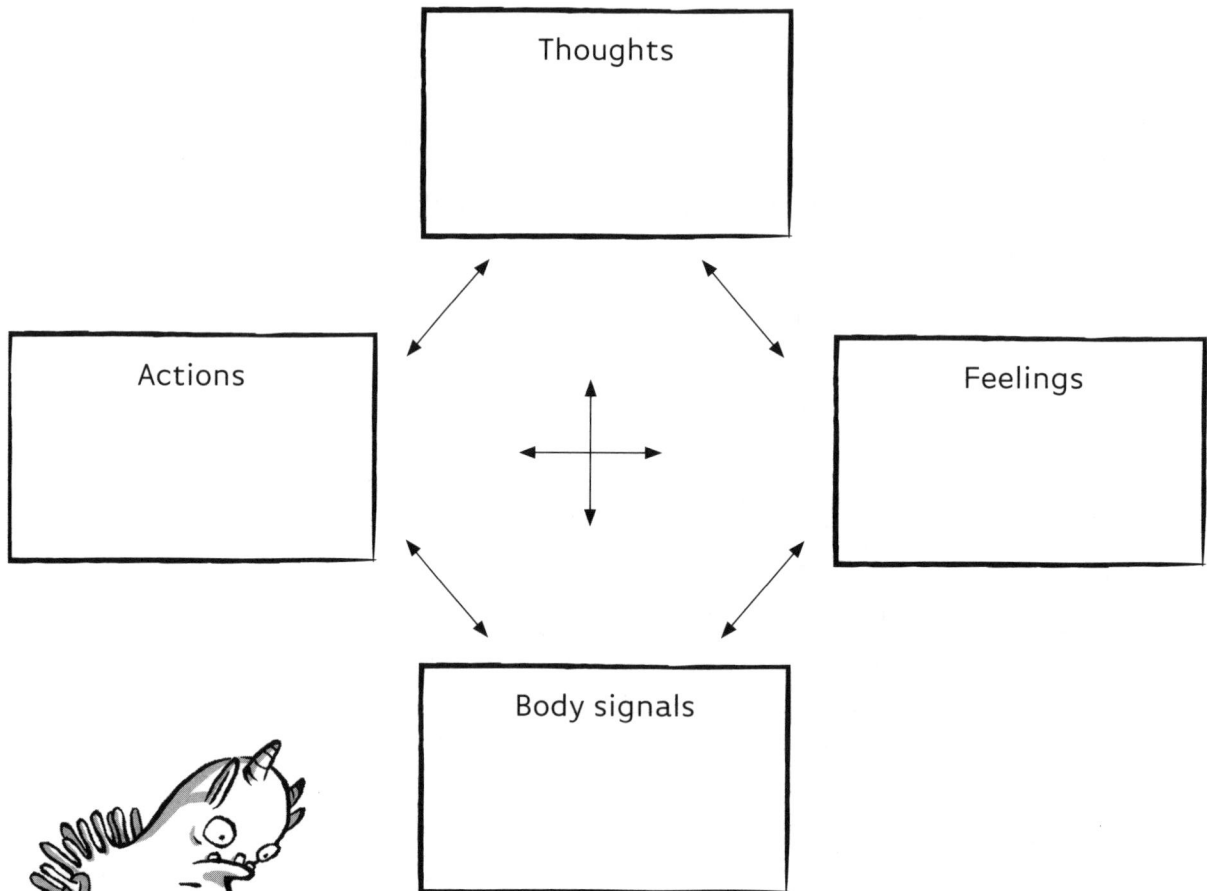

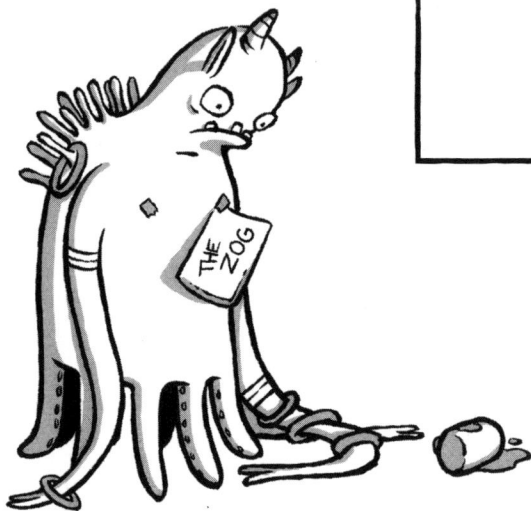

Thoughts

Actions

Feelings

Body signals

The Zog's thoughts, feelings, body signals and actions had all changed and become like a vicious cycle. The more worried and sad thoughts he had, the more upset he felt.

After some time, the Zog returned home. As he arrived he heard his Zen friends singing 'Happy Birthday' and calling his name. They had prepared a surprise party at his home. At this point, the Zog's sad and worried feelings started to change. He became happy and overjoyed. His tummy became calm and his body was relaxed. His thoughts also changed: 'Everyone remembered me', 'My friends care about me' and 'I love birthdays'. The Zog laughed and jumped up and down with excitement.

Notice how the Zog's thoughts, feelings, body signals and actions all changed once again.

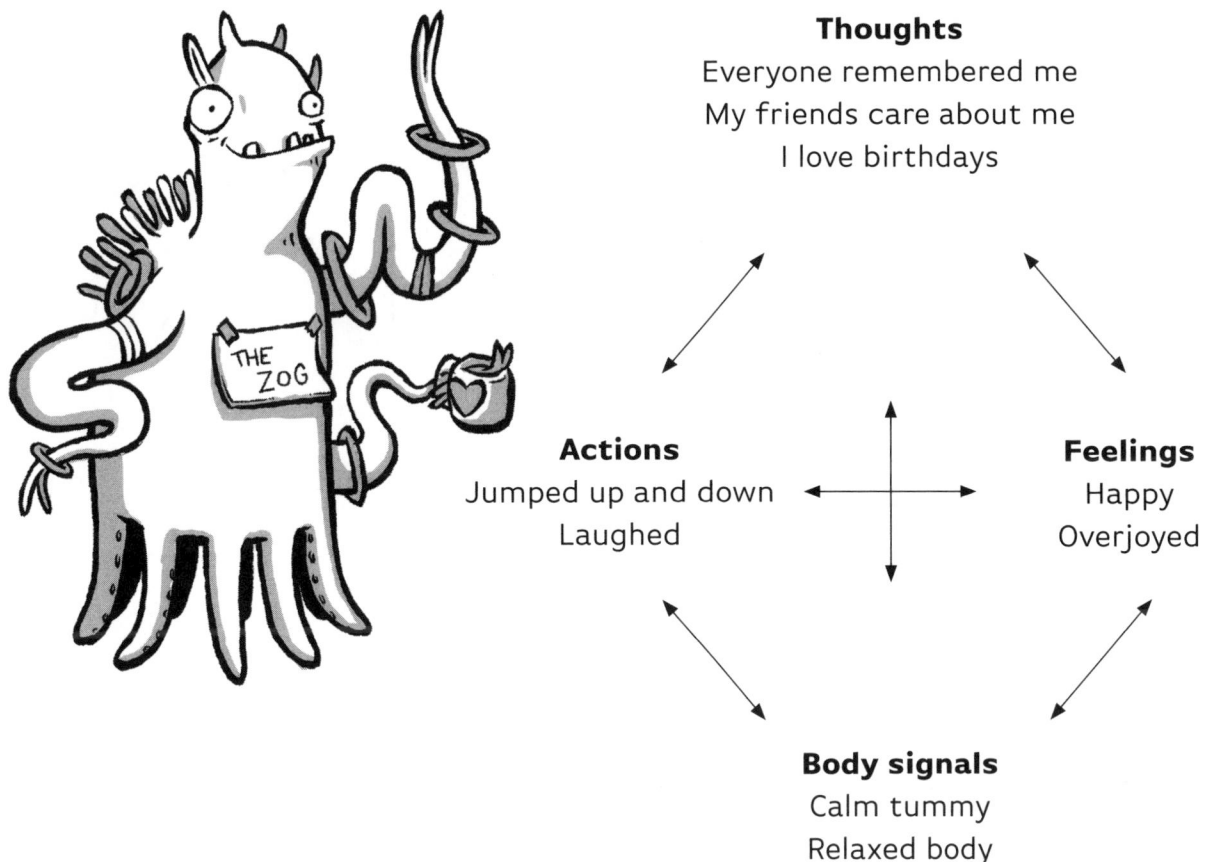

Thoughts
Everyone remembered me
My friends care about me
I love birthdays

Actions
Jumped up and down
Laughed

Feelings
Happy
Overjoyed

Body signals
Calm tummy
Relaxed body

Your actions

Sometimes when you feel sad you don't have as much fun doing the things you used to like doing. You give up on things faster, or get into more fights with family and friends. When you are scared you might have bad dreams or become more shy around people. You may also stay away from the things that scare you, for example dogs, school or lifts. Draw or list some of the cool connections between your actions and your scared and sad feelings.

Draw or write your actions or the things that you do when you are sad:

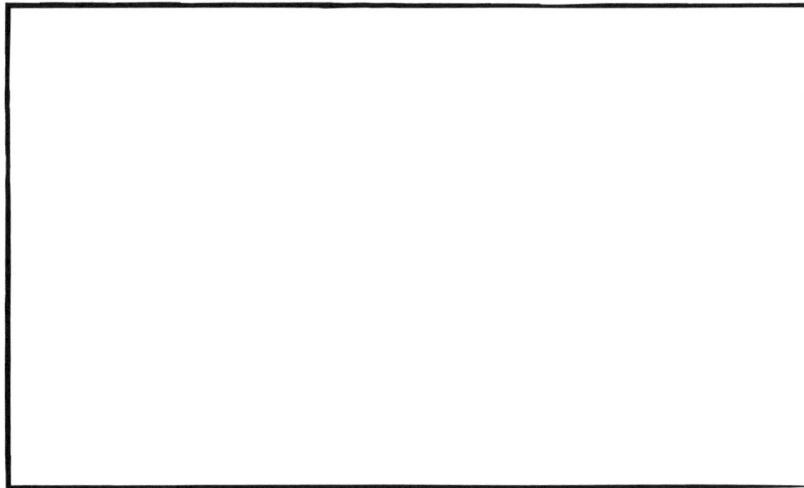

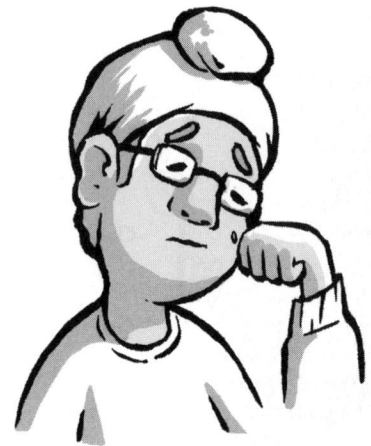

Draw or write your actions or the things that you do when you are scared:

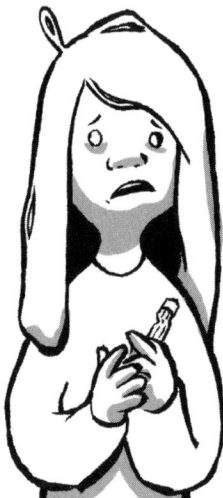

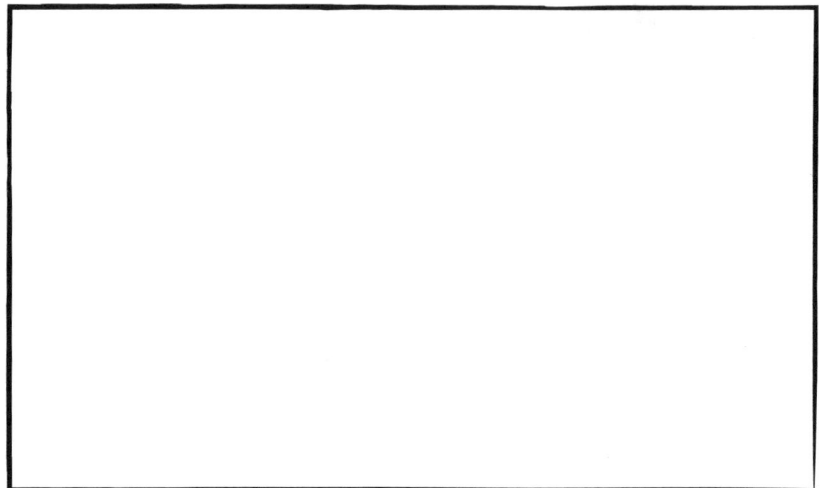

Different cool connections

Human beings can quickly change from one feeling to another, for example calm and happy to feeling angry, scared or stressed out. This is because we have a super-fast communication system in our brains which connects our thoughts, feelings, body signals and actions.

Situation

A child bumps into you in the school corridor. Notice how different people react to the same situation depending on their different thoughts and feelings.

Angry

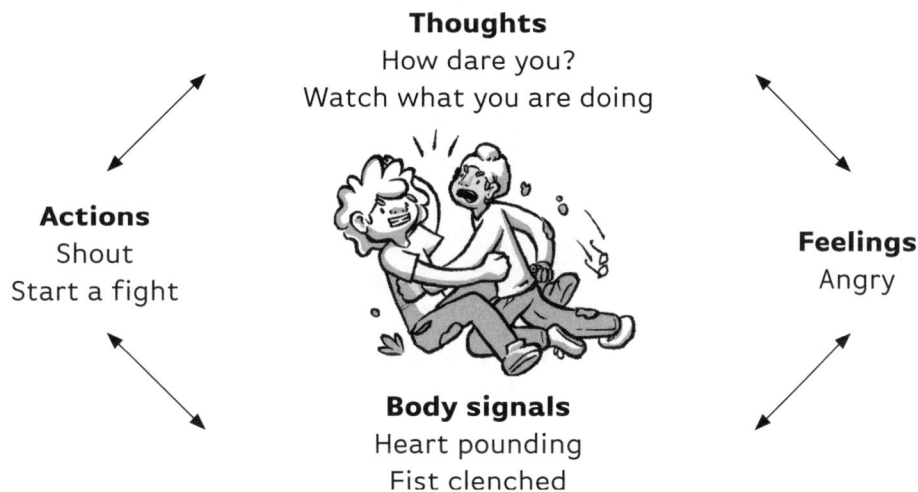

Thoughts
How dare you?
Watch what you are doing

Actions
Shout
Start a fight

Feelings
Angry

Body signals
Heart pounding
Fist clenched

Excited

Thoughts
Wow!
Amir bumped into me
It's because he likes me

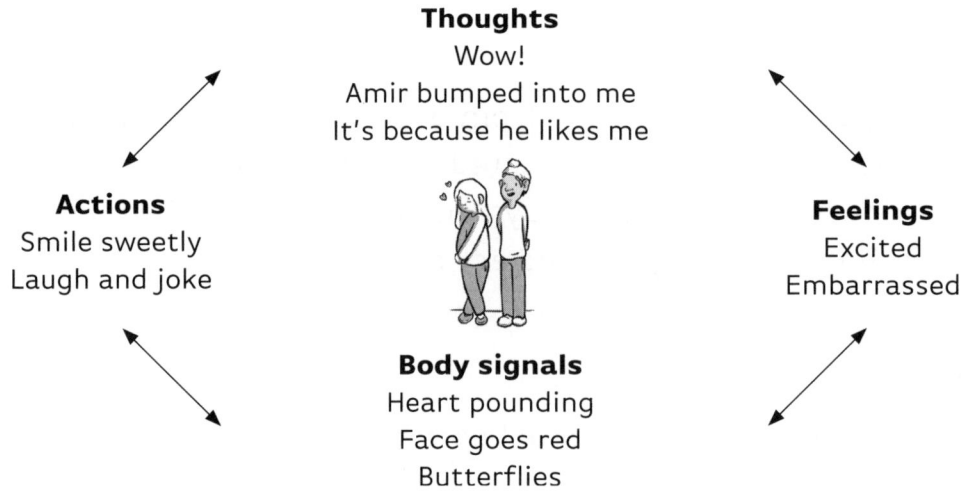

Actions
Smile sweetly
Laugh and joke

Feelings
Excited
Embarrassed

Body signals
Heart pounding
Face goes red
Butterflies

Worried

Thoughts
The poor girl
I need to help her

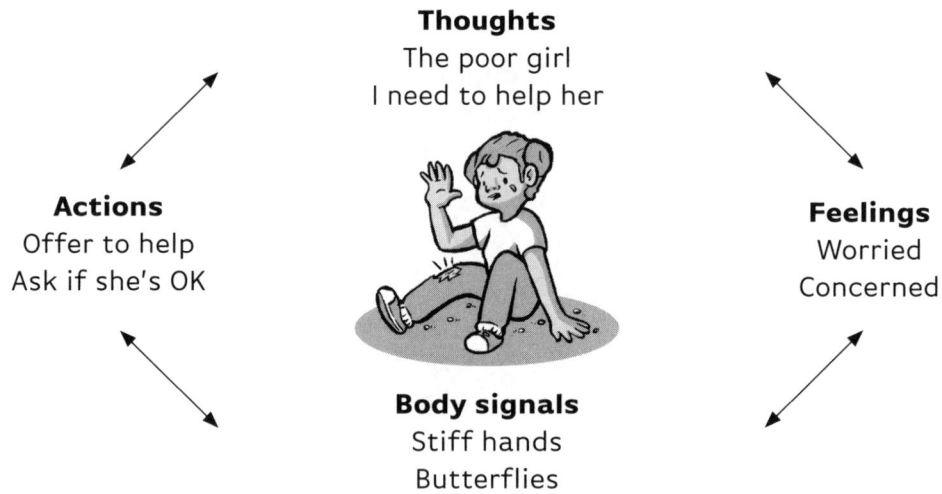

Actions
Offer to help
Ask if she's OK

Feelings
Worried
Concerned

Body signals
Stiff hands
Butterflies

Sad

Thoughts
I'm so stupid
No one likes me

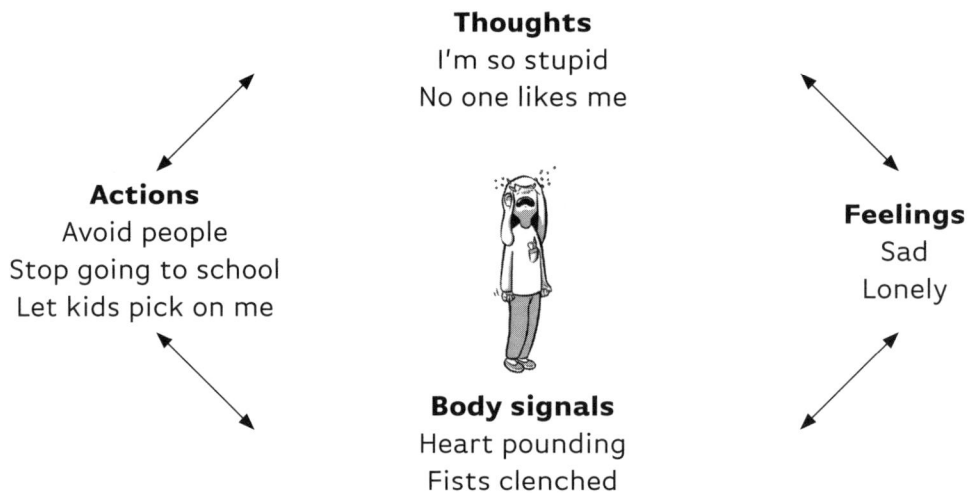

Actions
Avoid people
Stop going to school
Let kids pick on me

Feelings
Sad
Lonely

Body signals
Heart pounding
Fists clenched

Cool connections example

What happened?

My mum and dad were shouting at each other last night. Mum ended up walking out and slamming the door.

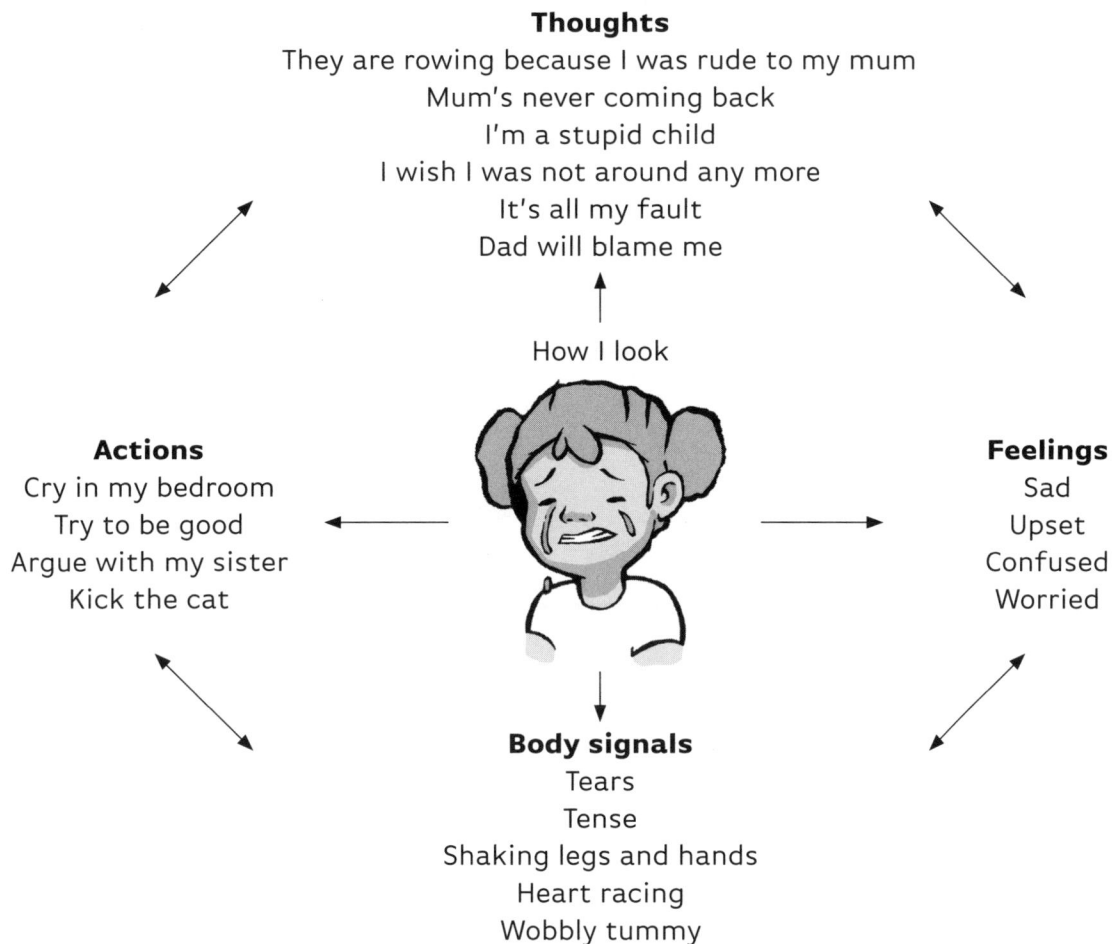

Thoughts
They are rowing because I was rude to my mum
Mum's never coming back
I'm a stupid child
I wish I was not around any more
It's all my fault
Dad will blame me

How I look

Actions
Cry in my bedroom
Try to be good
Argue with my sister
Kick the cat

Feelings
Sad
Upset
Confused
Worried

Body signals
Tears
Tense
Shaking legs and hands
Heart racing
Wobbly tummy

From the cycle above you can see that Katie is very upset about the row her parents had last night. Notice how her thoughts, feelings, body signals and actions are all connected with each other. Katie is clearly upset about her parents rowing. However, until she completed the cycle above, she was totally unaware of what thoughts and body signals were making her feel so unhappy and causing her to cry and lash out at others. Looking at the completed cycle has helped Katie to see the situation differently and explore her feelings more clearly.

My cool connections

Now it's your turn. First think of a time you were frightened and then a time you were sad before completing the boxes. Make cool connections by drawing how your face looked in the centre of each cycle.

I felt frightened when:

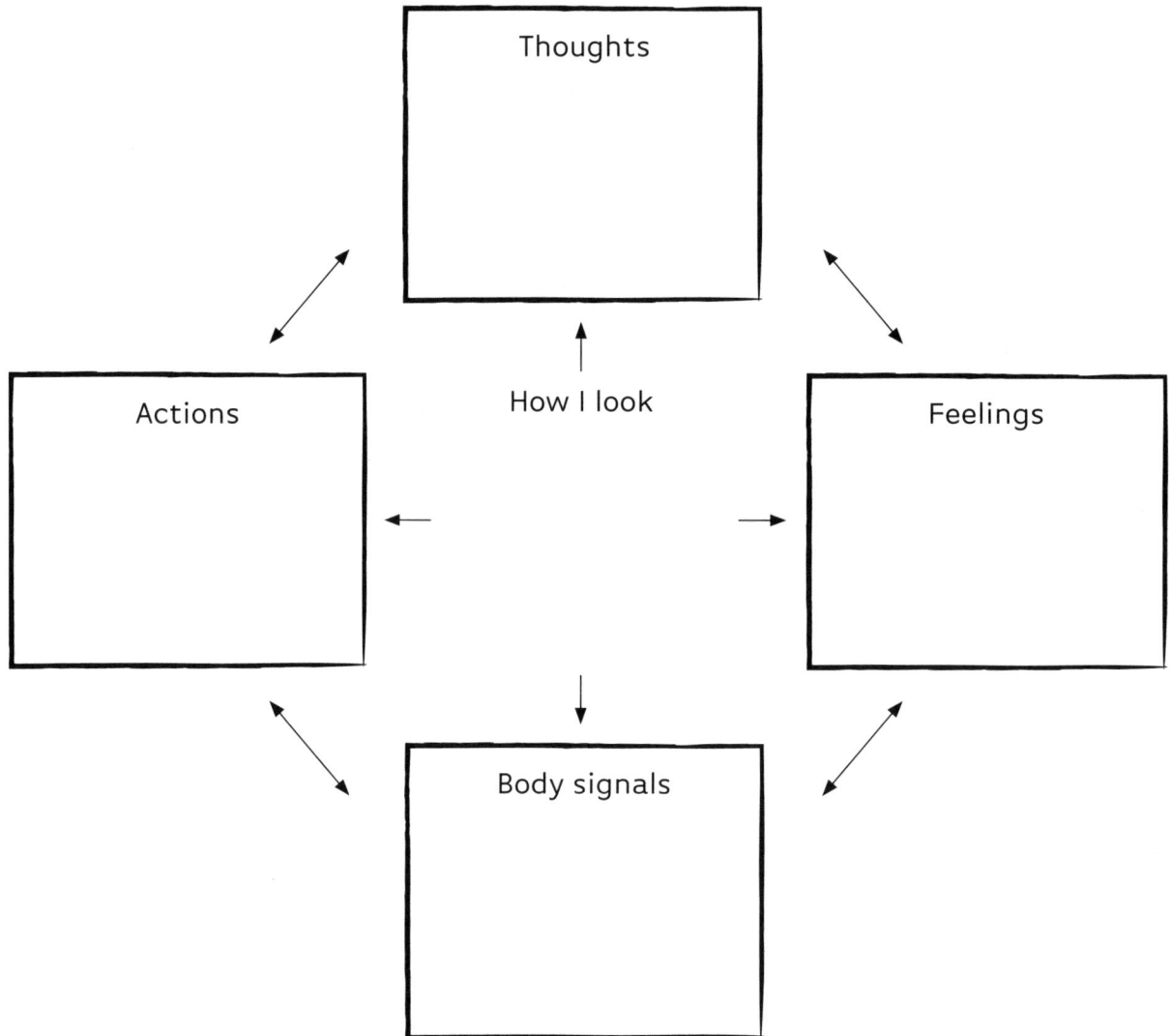

Thoughts

Actions

How I look

Feelings

Body signals

I felt sad when:

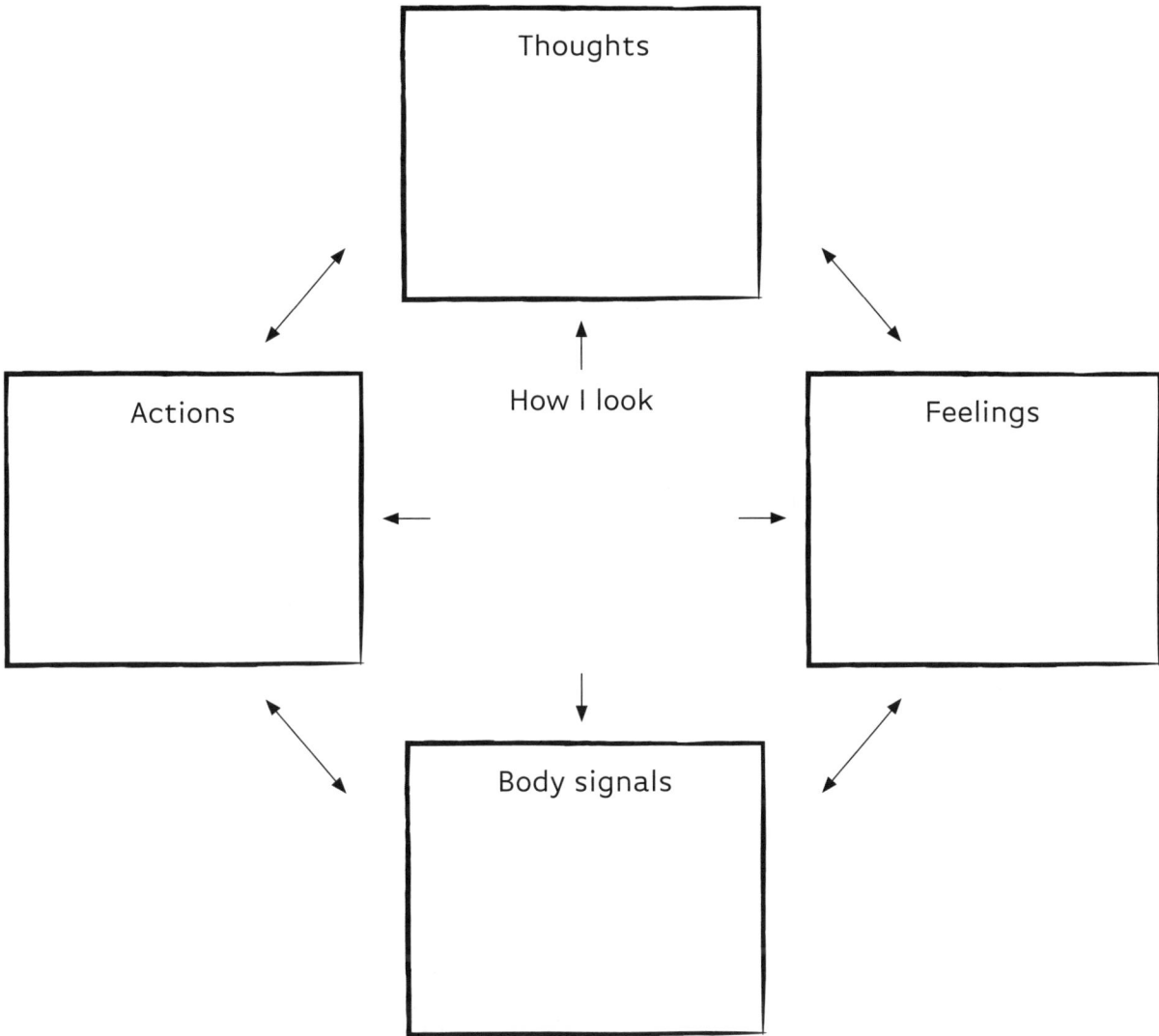

Thoughts

How I look

Actions

Feelings

Body signals

Cool connections game

This game is a further example of how your thoughts, feelings, body signals and actions are all connected.

How to play

- Find four pieces of paper or card. On each separate sheet write one of the following words:

  THOUGHTS   **FEELINGS**   **BODY SIGNALS**   **ACTIONS**

- Stick one piece of paper to each of the four walls in the room.

- The facilitator reads out the list on the following page. When the group members recognise thoughts, feelings, body signals or actions from the sentences, they must run to the associated part of the room. For example, if the facilitator reads 'Mary was feeling really sad', the group run to the area of the room marked 'feelings'.

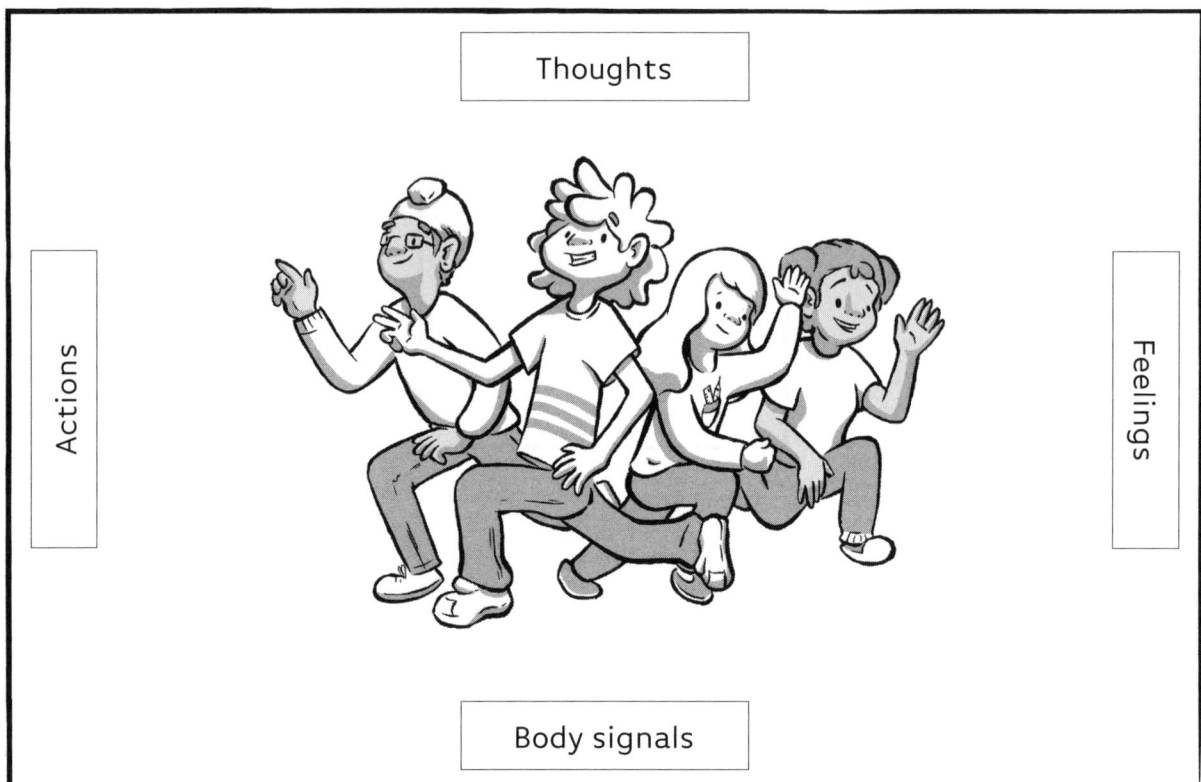

The game

- The Cool Connections Programme makes us feel so *happy*.

- Some boys at school took my lunch money and I thought, *'How dare they – I'm going to tell a teacher.'*

- I went to the dentist and looked up at the drill. *My heart started to pound in my chest.*

- The old lady saw a spider on the wall in her bedroom. She was so shocked that she *ran out of the room screaming.*

- The lion escaped from its cage at the zoo. I was so scared I started to *panic.*

- *'Help, help, help,'* thought the caretaker as he slipped on the wet floor.

- The girl stuck chewing gum on her chair at school. She started to feel quite *sick* when she noticed the head teacher looking at her.

- The boy *ran away* when he saw the bullies coming towards him.

- The girl found her maths test very *frustrating.*

- The children enjoyed the games so much that they thought, *'We'd like to play that again.'*

Home activity 6a: Quick quiz

In the box below, practise making cool connections by ticking whether the statements in the box on the left are thoughts, feelings, body signals or actions.

	Thought	Feeling	Body signal	Action
'I hate being away from my friends'				
Shaking				
Kicking a ball				
Tired				
'I really like pop music'				
'Oh no, here come those feelings again'				
Angry				
Sick				
Dizzy				
Climbing over the fence				
Frustrated				
'The teachers are so cool'				
Running				
Playing football				
'My fingers have gone tingly'				
Sweating				
'I love my clothes'				
Worried				
'It's driving me mad – I just can't cope'				
Upset				

Home activity 6b: Cool connections

Notice a time this week when you have had a strong feeling and then complete the boxes below. This could be a time when you have felt worried, upset, angry or sad. Write briefly what happened in the box before completing your cool connections (e.g. Amir bullied me at school, or my mum told me off). Draw what your face looked like in the centre of each cycle.

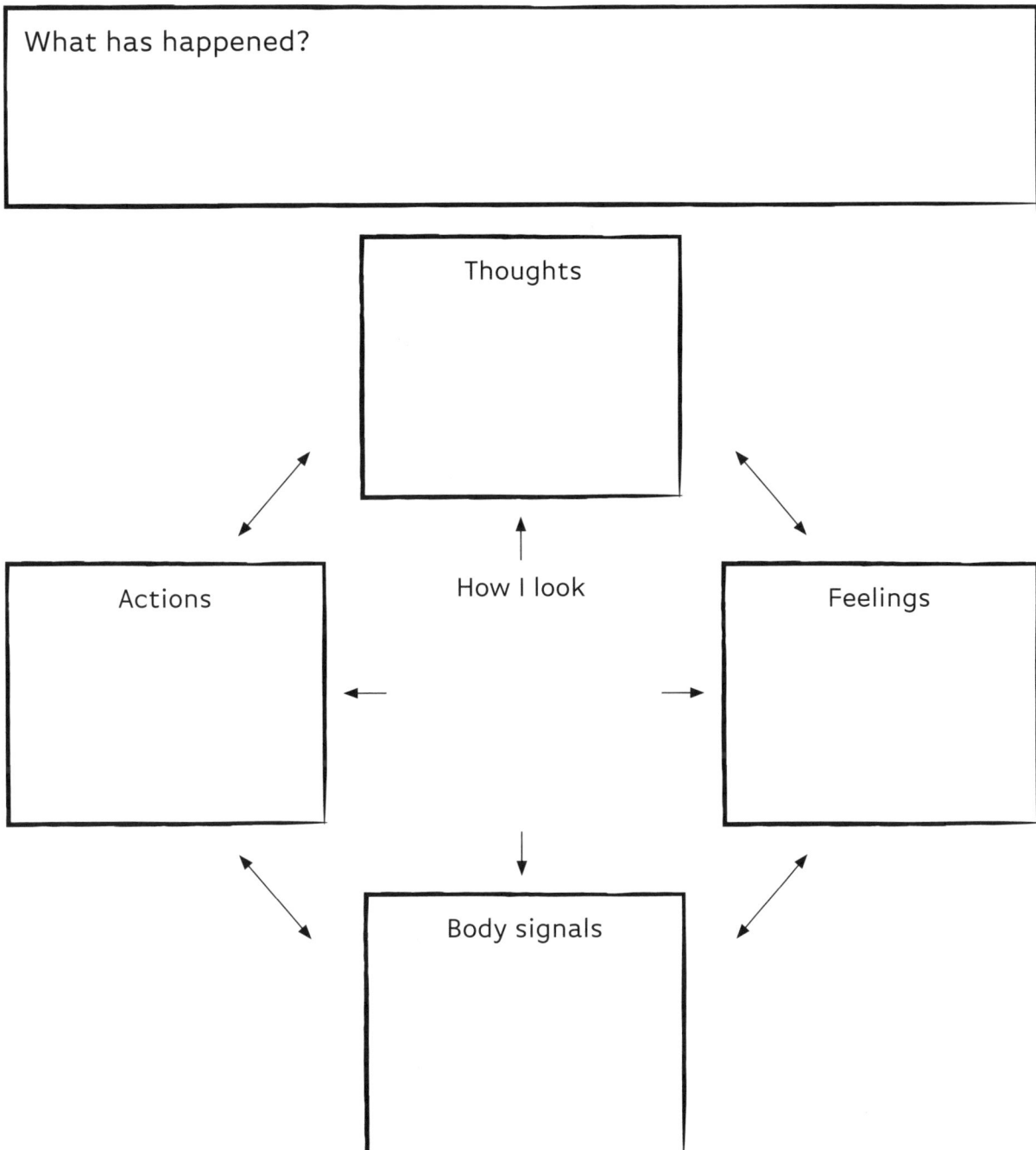

What has happened?

Thoughts

How I look

Actions

Feelings

Body signals

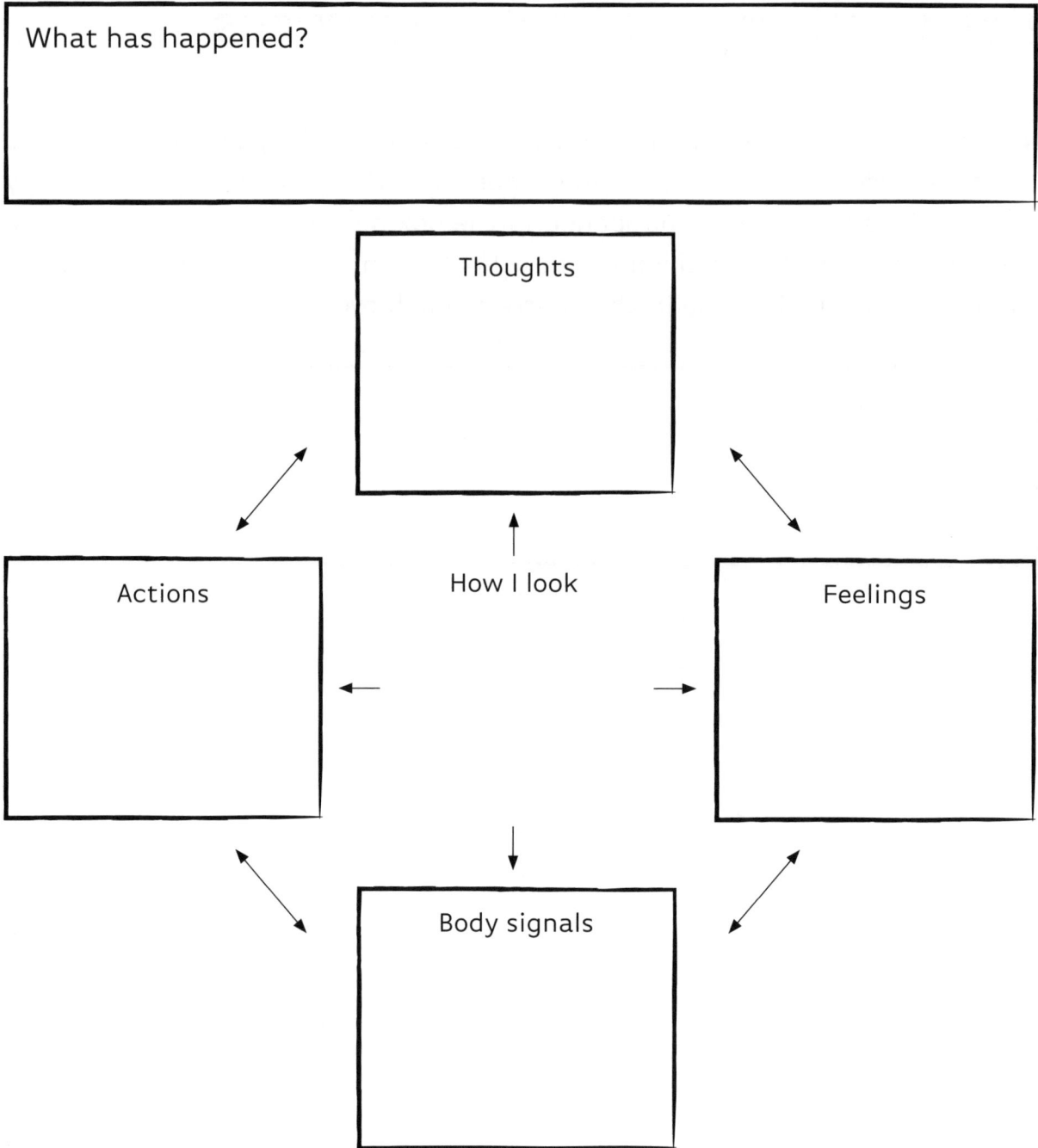

What has happened?

Thoughts

How I look

Actions

Feelings

Body signals

SESSION 7: TYPES OF THINKING

Aims and objectives

- Learn that there are different ways of thinking and that these can affect how we feel and act.

- Learn questions which help us understand in more detail what is upsetting us.

Materials

Chairs, pencils, cap or hat for 'The gloomies' exercise (not essential). Selection of hand or finger puppets.

Agenda and tips for running the session

Exercises in bold in the left-hand column should be included in both long and short sessions. Other exercises are optional and can be included in groups where there is more time. Many fun activities and games are included as optional. Despite sometimes being short of time it is important not to cut all the 'fun' out of the programme or you will lose the children's enthusiasm.

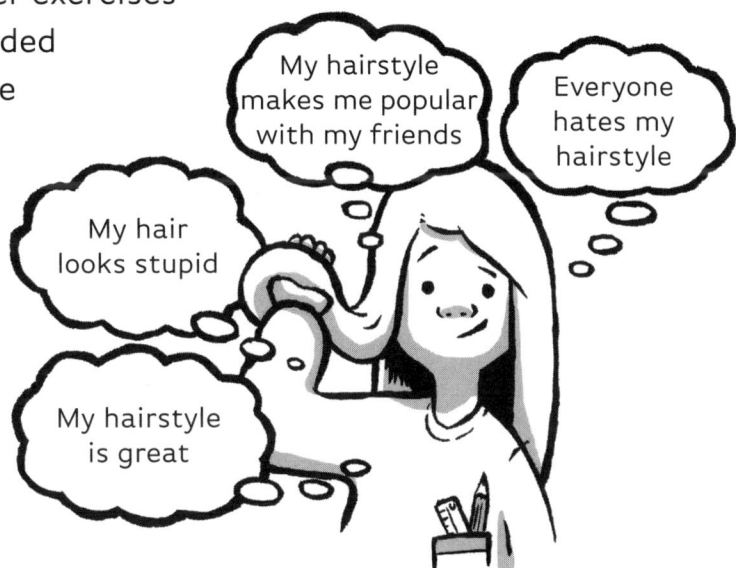

My hairstyle makes me popular with my friends

Everyone hates my hairstyle

My hair looks stupid

My hairstyle is great

Short session

EXERCISE	COMMENT
Feedback	Welcome the children and share agenda for session with the group. Obtain brief feedback from the children's week.
Review Home activities 6a and 6b	Children can briefly share their work. Facilitators collect home activities to explore in more detail after the session and return the following week or at the end of the programme.
'Get knotted'	Fun way to start the session. If children are reluctant to hold hands they can hold jumper or shirt sleeves or wrists.
The beautiful hag	Children are encouraged to feed back on the pictures. It is emphasised that there are no right or wrong answers. It is interesting how different children perceive the pictures. We have noticed that negative thinkers often see the old hag first and the two faces as aggressive. Children with a more positive outlook tend to observe the beautiful lady first and suggest seeing two lovers/friends.
Are you a Pollyanna?	Children are encouraged to choose to read the different parts. You may wish to include puppets for this exercise.
The gloomies	We have noticed that children who feel unhappy about themselves are often particularly good at this exercise. A cap or hat can be worn by the gloomy thinker at the discretion of the facilitators.
Downward diggers	Children are asked to volunteer a couple of the characters they have placed in each box. Children may also be asked in which box they would place themselves.

My downward digger | Children find using puppets good fun and the children can hide behind the puppet characters they have chosen. Some facilitators may prefer not to use puppets and would rather use a different tool for the exercise. For example, children could dress up, wear different hats or draw the answers using speech bubbles. This exercise can sometimes make children feel low, especially if they connect the puppet's worry or upset with themselves. Other group members can be encouraged to offer support and/or help with this. See Notes below.

Or

Helping hands | Some children may have difficulty identifying people they can trust to support them or have difficulty thinking of activities they enjoy doing. This can be an indicator that the child is experiencing low mood or depression. On these occasions, facilitators should empathise with the individual and invite the other group members to offer their support. Following the group, a network should be developed either by facilitators or teachers to provide support for the child. Buddy groups, school prefects or mentors can be useful here. Also, children can be encouraged to get involved in inside or outside school/activity groups.

Wise worriers | This is a helpful exercise, especially in reducing generalised anxiety (when children seem to have ongoing worries about everything all of the time). When children struggle with this exercise it may highlight high levels of anxiety or difficulties with problem-solving. In some cases, thinking about themselves having these anxiety-provoking scenarios may feel too threatening. Instead, the child should be encouraged to write what a friend would do in the scenarios.

Home activity 7: Eavesdropping | Children gain an awareness of different types of thinking. This can help normalise their own experiences and develop alternative ways of thinking.

Long session

Include 'Get knotted', 'Downward diggers', 'My downward digger', 'Helping hands' and 'Wise worriers'. More time can be spent with 'The gloomies' 'Downward diggers', 'Helping hands' and 'Wise worriers'. Children can act out an example of a positive thinker or negative thinker. We found it useful to show a clip from the film *Pollyanna*. The children can be asked what they notice about the effect Pollyanna's 'Glad game' and general attitude to life have on the people around her.

Notes

We are not aiming to help children become positive thinkers instead of negative thinkers. Rather we are helping children to become aware of the effect different types of thinking can have on their feelings, body signals and actions. Children often have quite fixed 'black and white' ways of thinking. The first part of this session aims to introduce some 'shades of grey' and explore alternative ways of thinking about things. The 'Downward diggers' exercise is quite difficult and can cause children to become quite frustrated. However, the aim is to help children get to the heart of what is troubling them. Looking at the worst possible outcomes can help reduce anxieties in some children, while in others coping/problem-solving strategies are initiated. The 'Helping hands' and 'Wise worriers' exercises provide children with some basic ways to help cope with their fears and anxious thoughts. Some facilitators running short sessions may seek advice in choosing between 'Downward diggers' and 'Helping hands'/'Wise worriers'. As a guide, the 'Downward diggers' exercise is a useful tool for children who are frequently upset or anxious but remain unclear regarding the thoughts and beliefs which are maintaining these feelings. 'Helping hands' and 'Wise worriers' are useful for children who feel isolated or helpless and provide a useful strategy for coping with generalised anxiety or worries that feel 'out of control'.

'Get knotted'

- The group form a chain by holding hands or wrists.

- One end of the chain weaves his or her way under the arms of the other children in the chain to form a tangle.

- Without breaking the chain, the children need to find a way to untangle themselves.

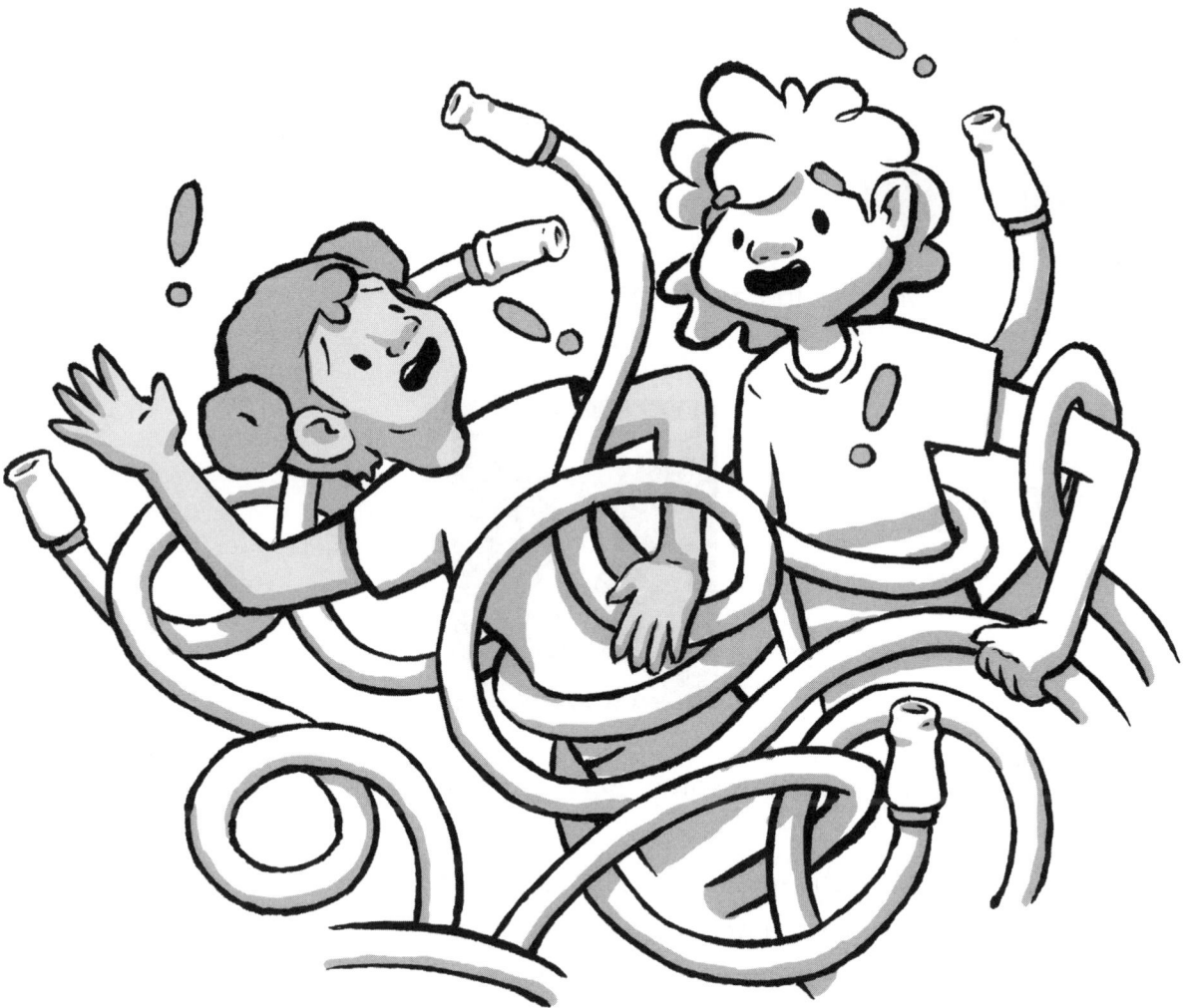

This exercise helps children to learn to work together and encourages problem-solving. Even if a problem is difficult to solve, by trying different ways you usually come to a solution in the end.

The beautiful hag

In the first picture below some people see an old hag while others see a young lady. The second picture can be seen as a vase or two faces looking at each other. Which do you see when you first look at the pictures? Tick or circle the boxes below:

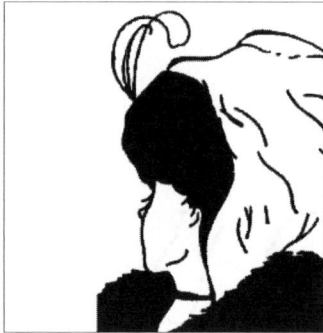

Old lady

Young lady

My Wife and My Mother in Law (1915). By W.E. Hill

Two faces

Vase

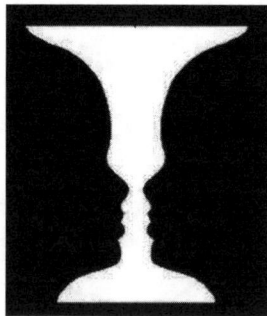

The Rubin Vase (1915). By E. Rubin

As you can see from these pictures, there is often more than one way of looking at things. There are no right or wrong answers, but the way we think about things does affect how we feel about them. For example, if you see an old hag in the first picture, you may feel afraid and look away from the picture. However, if you see the beautiful lady, you may feel happy and wish to meet her. In the second picture, some children say they see two angry people and feel upset. Others say they are two lovers staring into each other's eyes. Find out what others in your group feel about the pictures.

Are you a Pollyanna?

Because everyone is different, people often have quite different thoughts about things. Some people always seem to see the good or positive things in everything and everybody, while others only seem to see the bad or negative things in life. This is sometimes described as seeing a glass as half full or half empty.

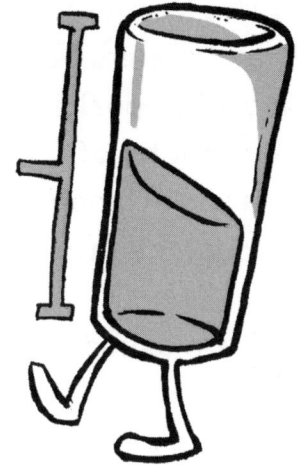

Pollyanna is a famous story about a little orphaned girl who starts her new life with a strict old aunt. To help her cope with her troubles, she plays a game which her father taught her called the Glad Game.

This involves finding a silver lining in every cloud. She tries to find a useful way of looking at things, even in the most unhappy situations in her life. Having such a positive outlook, Pollyanna soon finds that she becomes very popular, and playing the Glad Game seems to brighten up some of the unhappy characters she meets in the community she lives in.

Although trying to be positive is not always useful, you may find playing the Glad Game helps you to explore different ways of thinking about things, especially if you are feeling really stuck and unhappy. In the boxes below write the names of anyone you know who tends to think really negatively about everything, or like Pollyanna anyone you know who always seems to look on the bright or positive side of life.

Positive thinkers	Negative thinkers

The gloomies

With gloomy thinking we focus only on negative things that happen. We notice all the things that go wrong. Anything positive tends to get overlooked, disbelieved or thought of as unimportant. It is as though we are wearing a 'gloomy thinking cap' or that we see everything through negative glasses. See the examples below:

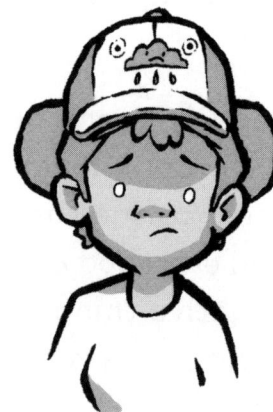

You are asked to go to a party with someone you really like.
You think, 'They probably couldn't find anyone else to go with. That's why they're asking me.'

Amir did well in his maths test.
He thinks, 'Oh well, it was an easy test. If it was harder I would be sure to fail.'

A friend tells Katie: 'Your hair looks lovely today.'
'She's only saying that because she wants me to help her. She thinks I look ugly really.'

The gloomy thinking cap challenge

A volunteer from the group puts on the 'gloomy thinking cap'. While they are wearing the cap, they can only see the negative or gloomy side of things. They see the worst in the world, themselves and everybody. The challenge is for other group members to try and make the person wearing the 'gloomy thinking cap' be cheerful and laugh or say something positive like Pollyanna. Each person in the group challenges the cap wearer with one question, a joke or a funny face. If the cap wearer laughs, smiles or says something positive, they have lost the challenge and someone else wears the 'gloomy thinking cap'.

Downward diggers

To understand what is upsetting you about a worry or problem, make some cool connections by using a 'downward digger' question. For example:

What is the worst thing about that?

Or

What is the worst thing that could happen?

It may seem simple, but with a little practice and the help of a downward digger question it is possible to dig right to the heart of a problem or worry and see why it upsets you so much. Knowing what is at the bottom of your worry can be a big step to overcoming your problem or understanding other people's. See the examples below and then make up a problem and have a go with a friend. Show your downward digger to the group.

Downward digger 1

My problem is that I am scared to talk out in class.

What is the worst thing that could happen if you had to talk in class?
I will make mistakes and stumble over the words.

And if that were true, what would be the worst thing about that?
Other kids will laugh at me.

And if other kids laugh at you, what would be the worst thing about that?
I will get really embarrassed and go very red.

What's the worst thing about going red?
I will look stupid.

What's the worst thing about looking stupid?
Kids in the class will think I'm stupid.

What's so bad about that?
I'll think I'm stupid.

Downward digger 2

My problem is maths in school.

What's the worst thing about maths?
I keep getting told off by my teacher.

What's the worst thing about that?
He gets really mad and shouts.

What's the worst thing that could happen?
I could get a detention.

What's the worst thing about that?
My parents might find out.

What's the worst thing about that?
They will get really upset with me.

What's the worst thing that could happen?
They will think I'm a bad kid.

What's the worst thing about that?
They will stop caring about me.

What's the worst thing that could happen?
I'll know I'm a bad kid.

And if you are a bad kid, what's the worst thing about that?
No one will like me and I'll end up sad and lonely forever.

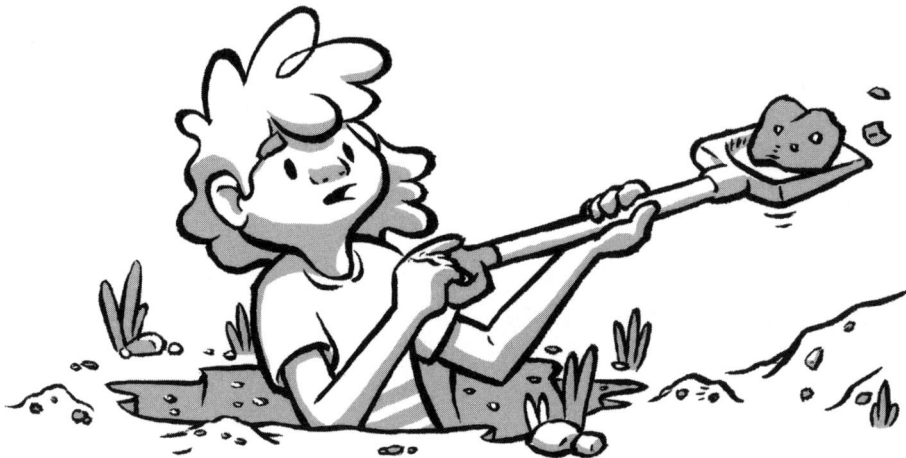

My downward digger

Choose a puppet to work with. Make up something that your puppet may be frightened or upset about and then write it in the box below. Make sure you only write one worry – rather than a complete story! For example, 'My puppet is worried that he has no friends', or 'My puppet is upset because he thinks he looks weird'.

After the downward digger, what thoughts were at the heart of your puppet's fears? Write some of the things that were most upsetting for the puppet in the box below. For example, your puppet may feel deep down that it is totally bad, stupid, ugly, useless, lonely. Use the puppet's own words to describe his or her feelings.

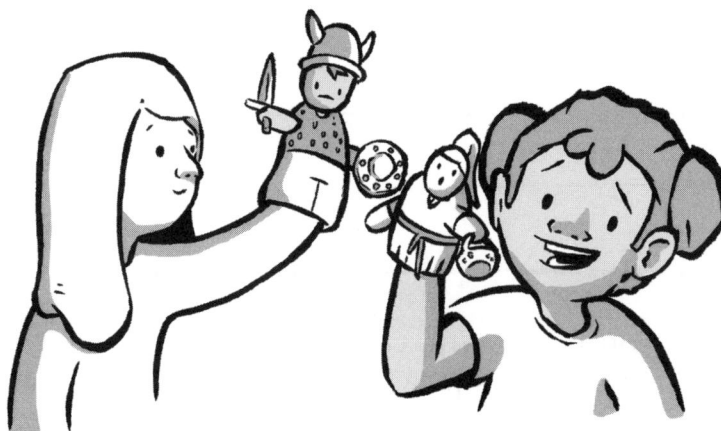

Helping hands

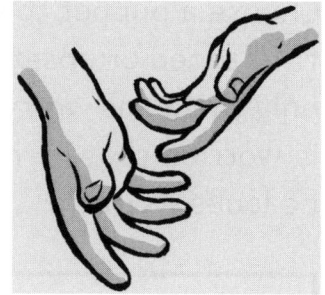

As you can see from the downward digger exercise, it is useful to become more aware of the thoughts which are making you feel gloomy or afraid. With this information you have more choice as to what to do next. Once you have caught yourself wearing a 'gloomy thinking cap' and have worked out your 'downward digger' thoughts, it is time to take action. It is not useful to let yourself spend too much time thinking over and over about your upset or worrying thoughts. Below are two actions you can take.

1. Talk to someone you trust about how you feel. Perhaps they could give you a 'helping hand'. This could be your parents, a family member, teacher or friend. Write the names of people who can support you in the box below.

2. You can also help yourself by doing something you enjoy. Sometimes when people feel upset they don't feel like doing anything at all. The truth is that if you don't do anything you are likely to feel more upset and very stuck. Get out and do an activity you enjoy and you will feel better much more quickly. In the box below, write some activities you enjoy doing and share them with the group. This could be football or swimming, drawing, painting, dancing and so on.

If you have time, you may want to experiment with the above idea. Try imagining yourself doing one of the activities you have written in the box above and see how it makes you feel.

Wise worriers

Often people have worrying thoughts which go round and round in their heads. The trouble is that the more worrying thoughts they have, the more worried and upset they feel. These thoughts usually start with 'what if' questions which often never get answered.

As well as talking to someone you trust and doing something you enjoy, a third way of helping yourself with worrying thoughts is to practise answering your 'what if' questions with 'then I can do' answers. It can calm you down and help you cope. You may also find this useful in helping your friends sort their worries out. Complete some of the questions below. Compare your answers with the rest of the group. In the blank row at the bottom, see if you can make up a 'what if' question and a 'then I can do' answer of your own.

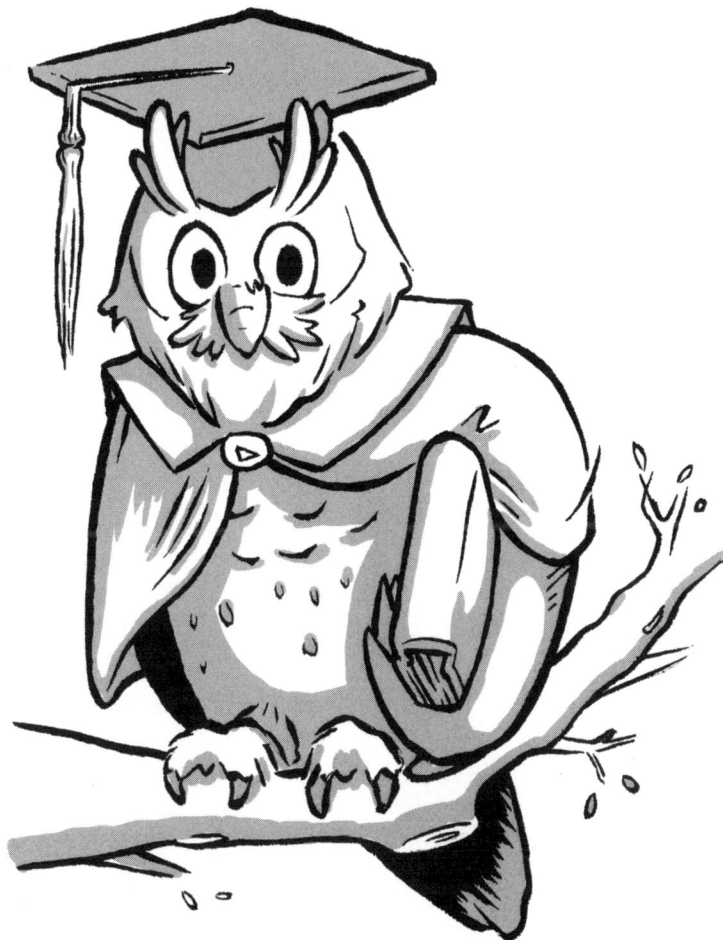

'What if' question	'Then I can do' answer
Example: What if I can't answer the questions in English today?	Then I can ask for help from my friend. Making mistakes is a good way to learn new things.
Example: What if I fall in the river while we are on holiday?	I can be prepared by wearing a life jacket. I will tell my friends I can't swim before we leave. I will shout and scream for help. Someone will save me. Lots of people are going to be around.
What if I make a mistake in my school work?	
What if I get bullied at school? The bullies are so big.	
What if I cry in public? It will be so embarrassing.	
What if I get a serious illness?	
What if someone I care about gets attacked or dies?	

Home activity 7: Eavesdropping

Listen to your friends, family and teachers this week and see if you can spot them talking as though they are wearing a 'gloomy thinking cap' or speaking like Pollyanna in her Glad Game (see 'Are you a Pollyanna?'). Briefly write who said what in the table below.

Child = C Adult = A	Pollyanna = P Gloomy = G	What did they say?
Example: A	G	No one ever hands in their homework.
Example: C	P	I learn something new every day.

SESSION 8: EXPLORING THOUGHTS

Aims and objectives

- Learn how to explore alternative ways of looking at your difficulties.

- Become 'scientific' in your approach to problem-solving by looking for evidence and facts rather than myths and speculation.

- Observe how 'green-light thoughts' can improve how you feel.

Materials

Chairs, pencils.

Agenda and tips for running the session

Exercises in bold in the left-hand column should be included in both long and short sessions. Other exercises are optional and can be included in groups where there is more time. Many fun activities and games are included as optional. Despite sometimes being short of time it is important not to cut all the 'fun' out of the programme or you will lose the children's enthusiasm.

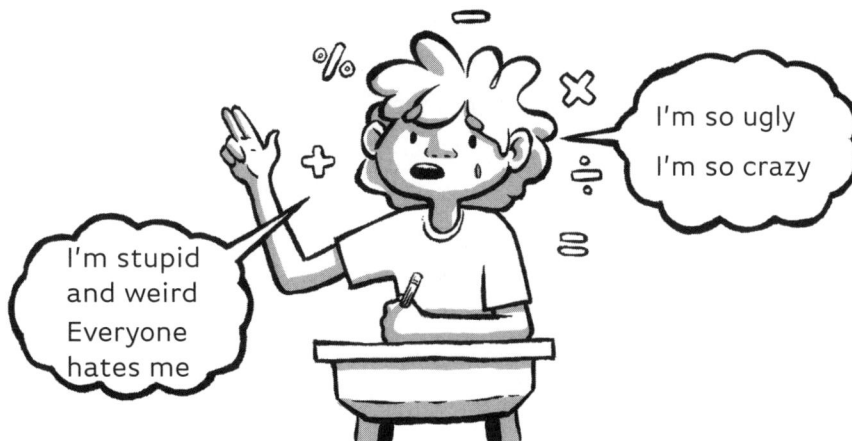

Short session

EXERCISE	COMMENT
Feedback	Welcome the children and share agenda for session with the group. Obtain brief feedback from the children's week.
Review Home activity 7	Children can briefly discuss their findings following the eavesdropping exercise. What did they notice? Facilitators collect home activities to explore in more detail after the session and return the following week or at the end of the programme.
Thought–feeling cool connections	Encourage children to make the connection between their thoughts and the way they feel. Children can be asked to share one answer with the rest of the group. If the children make different connections from the rest of the group this can be discussed openly in a non-judgemental way.
Traffic light thinking	Makes a link between different types of thinking and a traffic light system. Children do not need to focus too much on amber thoughts (observational-type thoughts). However, they have been included to help prevent children exploring their thoughts in 'black and white' or inflexible ways. For example, green thoughts are 'good' and red thoughts are 'bad'.
Red light, green light	Children write red- and green-light thoughts in the thought bubbles. There are no right or wrong answers. Children share the contents of one of their thought bubbles with the group.
Red, amber, green	It is important that there is a noticeable difference between the way the swimmer behaves when the children are cheering and saying green-light thoughts and when they are booing or saying red-light thoughts. It can be useful to compare this exercise with how children often say red-light thoughts to themselves, for example 'You idiot' when making a mistake. How useful are the things we say to ourselves?

SESSION 8: EXPLORING THOUGHTS

Changing those red-light thoughts	Children are encouraged to share with the group an example of how they have changed a red-light thought to a more useful green-light thought.
Traffic lights thought contest	Read the example in the thought bubbles to the group. Children could use drawings, models or puppets. Children show their scenes to the group. The participants are asked how it felt to play the different parts. The group can be asked whether the red- or green-light thoughts were the most powerful, useful, calming and so on. This can be compared with how much or little the children listen to their own red-light thoughts.
Example: Red-light thought challenge	Read through the example. The children may wish to read it; however, this can take more time. Ask the children to compare this exercise with the traffic lights thought contest exercise.
Red-light thought challenge	Red-light thoughts described about other children are often thoughts which children have about themselves. However, this is not always the case. This exercise can sometimes make children feel low, especially if they struggle to find evidence against their red-light thoughts. Other group members can be encouraged to offer support and/or help with this. See the Notes on this session.
Home activity 8a: Thinking quiz	Children practise identifying unhelpful and helpful thoughts.
Home activity 8b: Red-light thought challenge	Children practise the exercise, which aims to help them explore different ways of thinking. Finding more useful ways of thinking should help improve the children's mood and reduce anxious, angry or helpless feelings.

Long session

Include the 'Red, amber, green' exercise. This can be changed to suit the group (e.g. the swimmer could be a climber or a runner). More time can be spent on the 'Traffic lights thought contest' exercise. Children can be invited to share examples of red- or green-light thoughts that have been said to them by teachers, friends and family. Clips from magazines could be cut out and the children can connect red- or green-light thoughts to the pictures and share these with the group.

Notes

The exercises in this session aim to help children further explore alternative ways of thinking about things. We have a tendency to believe the red-light thoughts that we say to ourselves and act as though they are true. Although in some cases they may be true, generally the red-light or negative things we say to ourselves are not 100 per cent fact. By catching our red-light thoughts, we begin to reflect on them and explore evidence of their accuracy. Research suggests that the more evidence (or green-light thoughts) we find to contradict our negative or red-light thoughts, the better we feel. The trouble with red-light thoughts is that, although they are often intended to help motivate or protect us, the outcome is usually that they end up making us feel unhappy, angry, worried, more self-critical and often very stuck. This then causes a vicious circle (red-light thoughts = unhappy feelings = more red-light thoughts). The 'Red-light thought challenge' is difficult and will take frequent practice.

Thought-feeling cool connections

In the last session, we made cool connections about different ways of thinking. Some people think in positive ways, like Pollyanna with her Glad Game, while others seem to wear their 'gloomy thinking caps' and see things in negative ways that seem to keep them stuck. Most people have a mixture of both types of thinking in different situations. However, when we get upset, angry or worried, it is common for us to put on our 'gloomy thinking caps' and assume the worst about ourselves, everything and everyone. In this session, we are going to make some more connections about our thinking. In this exercise, be cool and connect the following thoughts in the left-hand column with the feelings in the right-hand column.

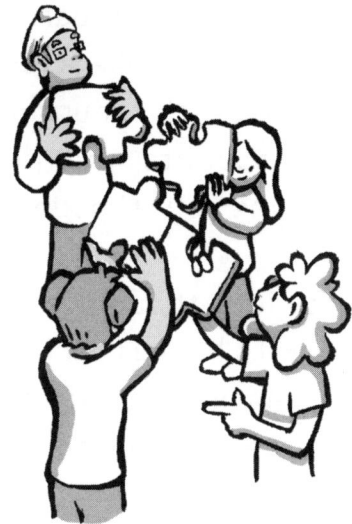

Thoughts	Feelings
I've got no friends because I'm a horrible person.	Happy
I can do it if I try.	Sad
I've coped with harder things than this before. The big wheel could be fun.	Angry
I want to hit all the other children at school.	Worried
I can always ask for help if I can't do it.	Confident
I just can't cope. It's just too hard.	Excited

Which do you think are the 'glad' thoughts, as in Pollyanna's Glad Game, and how can you tell?

Traffic light thinking

We have already learned cool connections about the way our thoughts affect our feelings. Like scientists, we are now going to explore the thoughts which connect with our upset, angry or worried feelings. We will begin by challenging the thoughts which keep us stuck. To do this, you may find it helpful to imagine your thoughts as the colours of a traffic light system.

Red-light thoughts usually make us feel more upset, worried or angry. They seem to hold us back and keep us feeling helpless and stuck in a vicious cycle. These thoughts often make us more aware of danger and the worst thing that can happen to us or other people.

Green-light thoughts are soothing or calming thoughts which make us feel better about ourselves and our situation. Green-light thoughts are useful and can help us cope better. These are 'doing' thoughts that help us take purposeful action towards achieving our goals.

Amber-light thoughts are noticing or observational thoughts. There is no positive or negative value placed on them. They are just thoughts that pop into our minds and then float off again, like a gentle breeze on a summer's day. Although amber thoughts may help us become more aware of things around us, they are less important in making the cool connections needed to help us explore the thoughts which cause us to feel so upset, worried or angry. If all thoughts were amber, we might well feel peaceful but we might also never get anything done. See the examples of traffic light thinking on the next page.

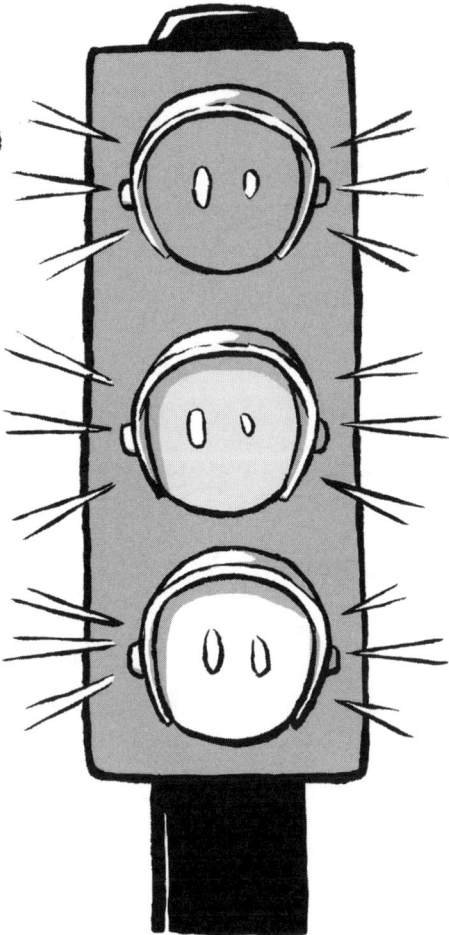

Red light, green light

Write a green-light thought and a red-light thought for each of the pictures with empty thought bubbles.

Example:

Green-light thought

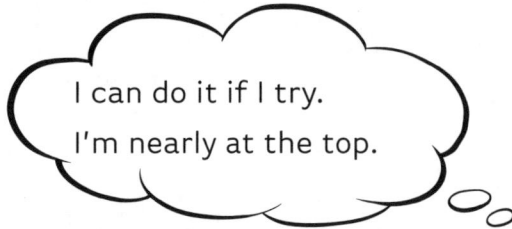

I can do it if I try.
I'm nearly at the top.

Red-light thought

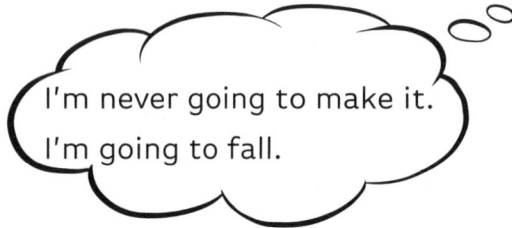

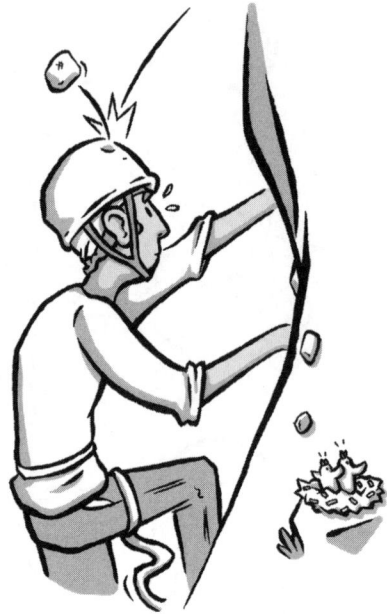

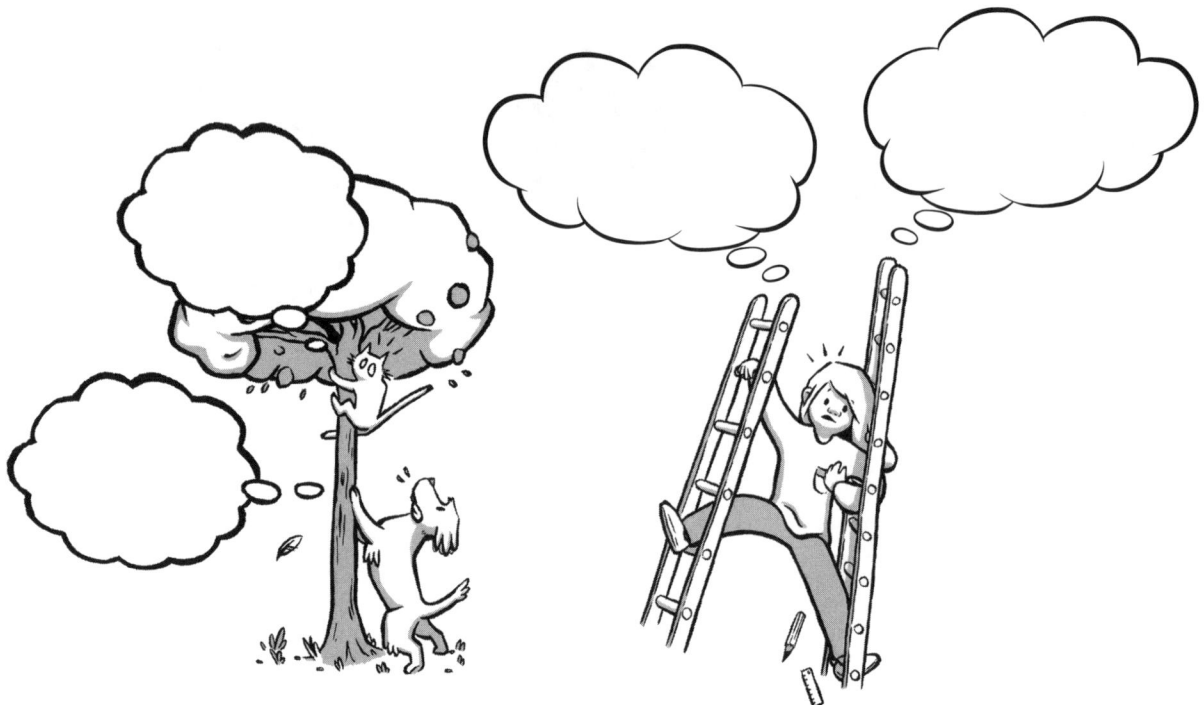

I'm never going to make it.
I'm going to fall.

Red, amber, green

The aim of this exercise is to experiment and see the effect our thinking can have on our actions. A volunteer from the group lies tummy downwards across a chair or a bench. They are asked to imagine that they are swimming in a race at the swimming pool. As the child pretends to swim, the rest of the group are encouraged to shout red-light thoughts such as 'You'll never make it' or 'You're so slow'. Following this exercise, the group members experiment by cheering and offering the swimmer green-light thoughts such as 'You are doing great' or 'Come on, you are nearly there'.

What effect did the red-light thoughts have on the swimmer?

. . . .

. . . .

What effect did the green-light thoughts have on the swimmer?

. . . .

. . . .

Give an example of an amber-light thought the swimmer may have had.

. . . .

. . . .

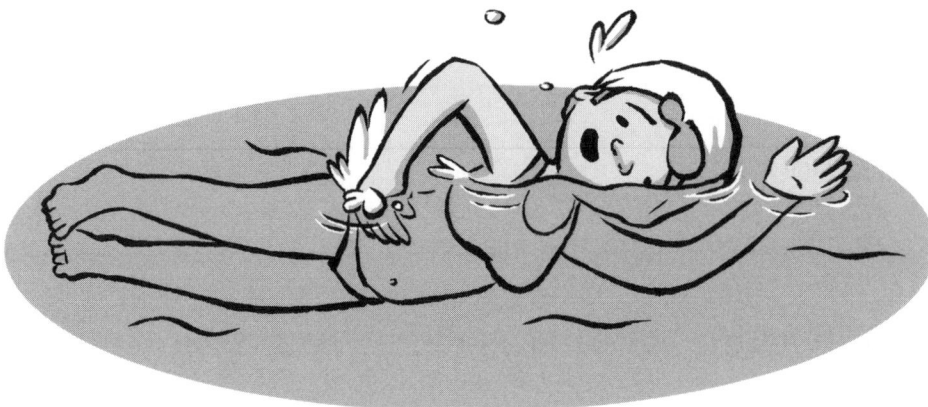

Changing those red-light thoughts

Choose two of the red-light thoughts below and see if you can change them into green-light thoughts.

Example

RED-LIGHT THOUGHT

'Everyone hates me because I'm so ugly. My hair is disgusting, my nose is too long and my legs are like bean poles.'

GREEN-LIGHT THOUGHT

'I know that I feel like I'm ugly sometimes but it doesn't mean that I really am. No one has actually said I'm ugly. Anyway, I am good at sports, English and music. My friends say I'm good company.'

Red-light thoughts

- I'll never be able to climb the mountain. It's just too high.

- There is no point in trying to join the sports team. They will only pick the good players and I never do well at anything.

- Donald and Daffy Duck keep picking on me. I'm never going back to that stupid duck school. It's 're-duckulous'. Everyone thinks I'm totally quackers.

- I'm feeling dizzy and sick again. Oh no, help, help, I'm probably going to die. No, please, not here in school. The other kids will see. I need my mum NOW. I feel dizzy. It's getting worse. Don't let me pass out and die. Arrrrrrh!

GREEN-LIGHT THOUGHT

. . . .

GREEN-LIGHT THOUGHT

. . . .

Traffic lights thought contest

Make a group of three with your friends and act out the following scene:

- *Person 1.* Act or draw a situation or goal that may be difficult for you to achieve. For example, climbing a mountain, reading out loud or confronting a bully.

- *Person 2.* Become Person 1's red-light thoughts. Try and stop Person 1 achieving the goal by saying negative thoughts to him or her. You may argue with Person 3 if you wish.

- *Person 3.* You have become Person 1's green-light thoughts. Try and help Person 1 achieve their goal by saying useful or calming thoughts to him or her. You may argue with Person 2 if you wish.

- Show your scene to the rest of the group. Discuss what effect the red- and and green-light thoughts might have on Person 1's feelings and actions.

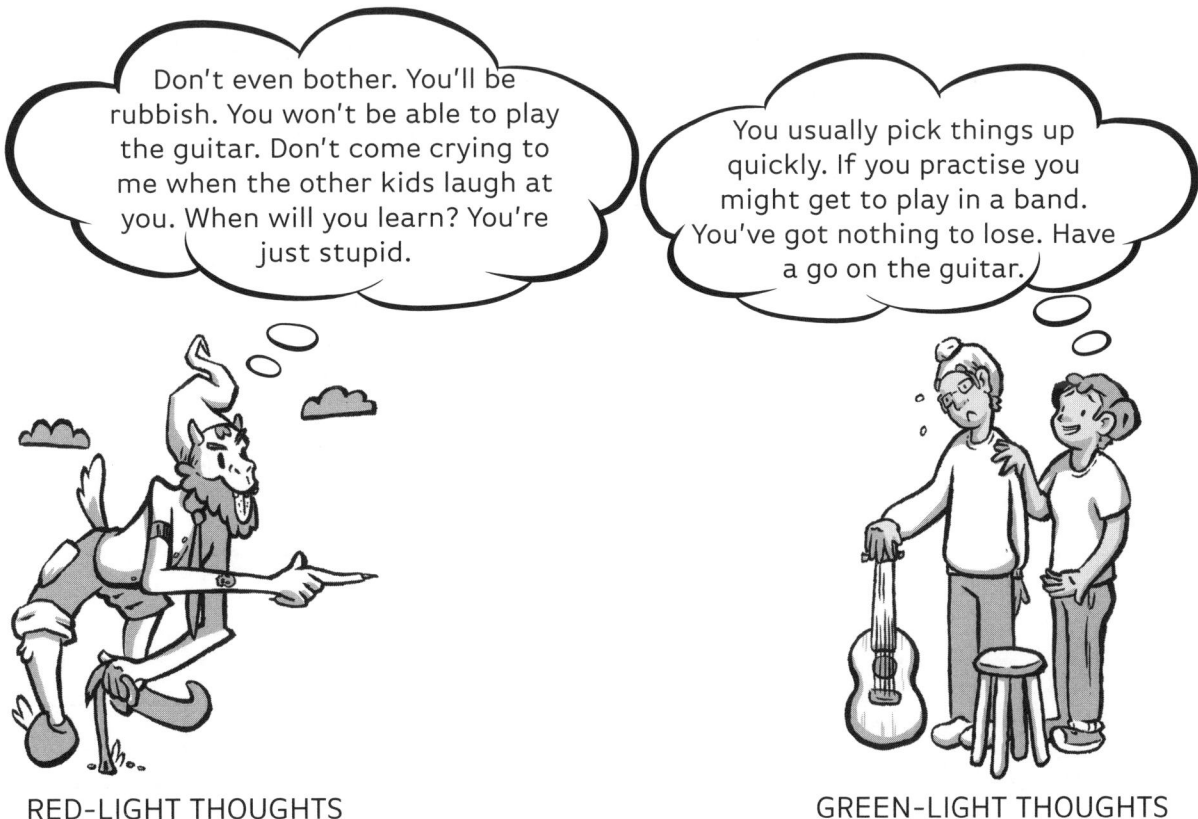

> Don't even bother. You'll be rubbish. You won't be able to play the guitar. Don't come crying to me when the other kids laugh at you. When will you learn? You're just stupid.

> You usually pick things up quickly. If you practise you might get to play in a band. You've got nothing to lose. Have a go on the guitar.

RED-LIGHT THOUGHTS   GREEN-LIGHT THOUGHTS

Example: Red-light thought challenge

Like a scientist looking for evidence, we are going to learn cool ways to test out thoughts which make us feel upset or worried. In the following exercise, think of a red-light thought that a friend might have about themselves. For example, 'I'm stupid' or 'No one likes me'. Having identified a thought, see if you can explore the evidence as shown in the example below. This is a red-light thought a friend might have about themselves:

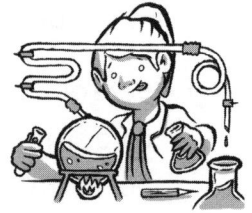

I am totally boring

How much on a score 0–10 do you think your friend believes their red-light thought?

Evidence which says my friend's red-light thought is 'completely' true	Evidence which says my friend's red-light thought is not 'completely' true
• His friends said that they could not go out with him at the weekend. • He had to stay at home on his own. • He does not like football like other kids. • Some kids at school call him a boffin. • He sometimes thinks that he does not fit in at school.	• No one has actually said that he is boring – only himself. • If he was boring, he would have no friends. Actually, he has got quite a few. • Lots of kids don't like football. It does not mean he is boring. Anyway, he does like snooker and fishing. • There are lots of other reasons why his friends may not be able to see him at the weekend – they may be grounded. • Everyone thinks they don't fit in sometimes. It does not always mean it is true.

How much on a score 0–10 do you think your friend believes their red-light thought now?

Red light thought challenge

Now it is your turn. Choose a red-light thought that you or someone else might have about themselves. Like a scientist, try and explore some green-light thoughts or more useful, calming thoughts to challenge the red-light thought. Don't forget to rate the thought both before and after challenging it. This is difficult – good luck!

Red-light thought you or a friend might have about themselves:

How much on a score 0–10 do you think you or your friend believe their red-light thought?

Evidence which says the red-light thought is 'completely' true	Evidence which says the red-light thought is not 'completely' true

How much on a score of 0–10 do you or your friend believe their red-light thought now?

Home activity 8a: Thinking quiz

Tick the boxes on the right to show green-light thoughts or red-light thoughts.

	Green-light thoughts	Red-light thoughts
I'm just totally stupid.		
They only want me to play because they can't find anyone else.		
I'm good at a lot of things, but if I'm not the best I always give up.		
They will all laugh at me if I go out dressed in these clothes.		
I can do it if I try.		
I'm so ugly.		
Someone will help me out if I get stuck.		
I won't bother going fishing on Saturday. I never catch anything anyway.		
I'm trying really hard with my homework because if I don't my mum will shout at me.		
If I am upset or worried I can tell people how I feel.		
I'm the best guitarist in the world.		
If I think about car crashes I might be in one.		
I hate school and everything about it.		
Some people like me and some don't – that's the way of the world.		
My worries make me feel like I'm going crazy.		
Just because I think there is a monster under my bed does not mean that there is.		
I'm totally rubbish at everything.		
I may not have done well this time but I really enjoyed taking part.		

Home activity 8b: Red light thought challenge

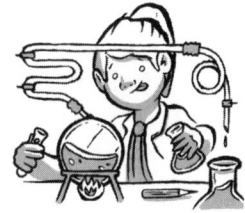

Next time you feel upset or worried, check out one of your red-light thoughts. Like a scientist, try and explore evidence for and against the red-light thought. After you have identified and rated your thought between 0 and 10, write down all the reasons why your red-light thought is true. Having done this, see if you can find any evidence to say that the thought is not true. This is difficult and can take a lot of practice. Don't give up – and good luck.

Red-light thought you have about yourself (I'm stupid, ugly, boring, etc.):

How much on a score 0–10 do you think you believe your red-light thought?

Evidence which says the red-light thought is 'completely' true	Evidence which says the red-light thought is not 'completely' true

How much on a score of 0–10 do you believe your red-light thought now?

SESSION 9: GOAL SETTING

Aims and objectives

- Make a six-point plan for goal setting.

- Encourage the group to work together and support each other through difficulties.

- Help the group to be clear and specific about their difficulties.

- Learn from watching others' goal setting.

Materials

Chairs, pencils, selection of hoops.

Agenda and tips for running the session

Exercises in bold in the left-hand column should be included in both long and short sessions. Other exercises are optional and can be included in groups where there is more time. Many fun activities and games are included as optional. Despite sometimes being short of time it is important not to cut all the 'fun' out of the programme or you will lose the children's enthusiasm.

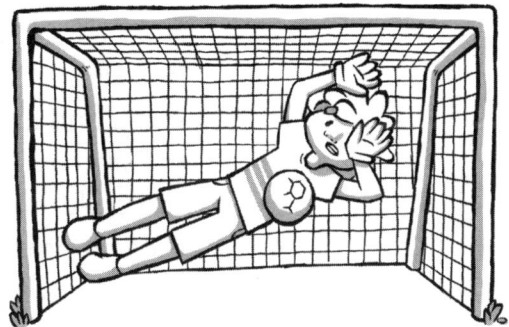

Short session

EXERCISE	COMMENT
Feedback	Welcome the children and share agenda for session with the group. Obtain brief feedback from the children's week.
Review Home activities 8a and 8b	Children can briefly discuss Home activities 8a and 8b. Facilitators collect home activities to explore in more detail after the session and return the following week or at the end of the programme.
Murder mystery	Children are encouraged to make connections between the skills required to find the murderer (observing others, listening, etc.) and the skills required for problem-solving and goal setting. Questions can be asked; for example, 'What did you need to do to catch the murderer?', 'How did you find out?', 'Which of your five senses did you use?', 'What happened if your guess was incorrect?'
IT solutions	This exercise is similar to the above. Some older groups of children may prefer this activity.
As clear as mud	Encourage the children to read the different parts of this exercise. Ask different children to share their answers with the group.
Hoola hoola	You will need a clear space to complete this exercise (sports hall or playground). The children find a partner. They are then given a hoop and asked to complete the exercise stages A–F before feeding back to the group. It is important that children work together, generating ideas and exploring possible consequences in sections A–D before putting their ideas into practice. Time is given for the children to practise and change their plan before the race commences. Following the race, children are asked to report back to the group about their outcomes. If facilitators prefer, a balloon or ball could be used instead of a hoop.

Home activity 9a: Superstars	It is useful to observe how other people cope with problems. Children learn a lot about coping with problems by observing others with good coping skills.
Home activity 9b: Goal setting	Children practise the exercise they have learned on pages 181–182.

Long session

Include 'IT solutions'. 'Superstars' can be incorporated into the main session rather than as a home activity exercise. Either in addition or as an alternative, a secret treasure (pieces of fruit or small sweets) can be hidden round the room while the children have their eyes closed. The children are then given a limited time to find the treasure and return to their seats. The children are asked what they did in order to find the treasure (listening, trying one place then another, watching others, etc.). The 'Hoola hoola' game can be extended either by providing every child with their own hoop or by dividing the group in half and having one hoop per team. If you have the time, short stories or online clips demonstrating good problem-solving or goal-setting skills can also be included. Some discussion about family members, friends or famous people who are good at solving problems or setting goals, and why, may also be helpful.

Murder mystery

- One child volunteers to be a detective. He or she is asked to leave the room while the other group members decide who will act as a murderer.

- The murderer kills his victims by winking at them. Should group members be winked at by the murderer, they should pretend to die 'loudly' and lie on the floor as if they were dead.

- When all members of the group are ready, the detective is invited back into the room. He or she must use detective skills to identify who the murderer is.

- When the murderer is found, the game is ended. You may wish to swap roles and play again.

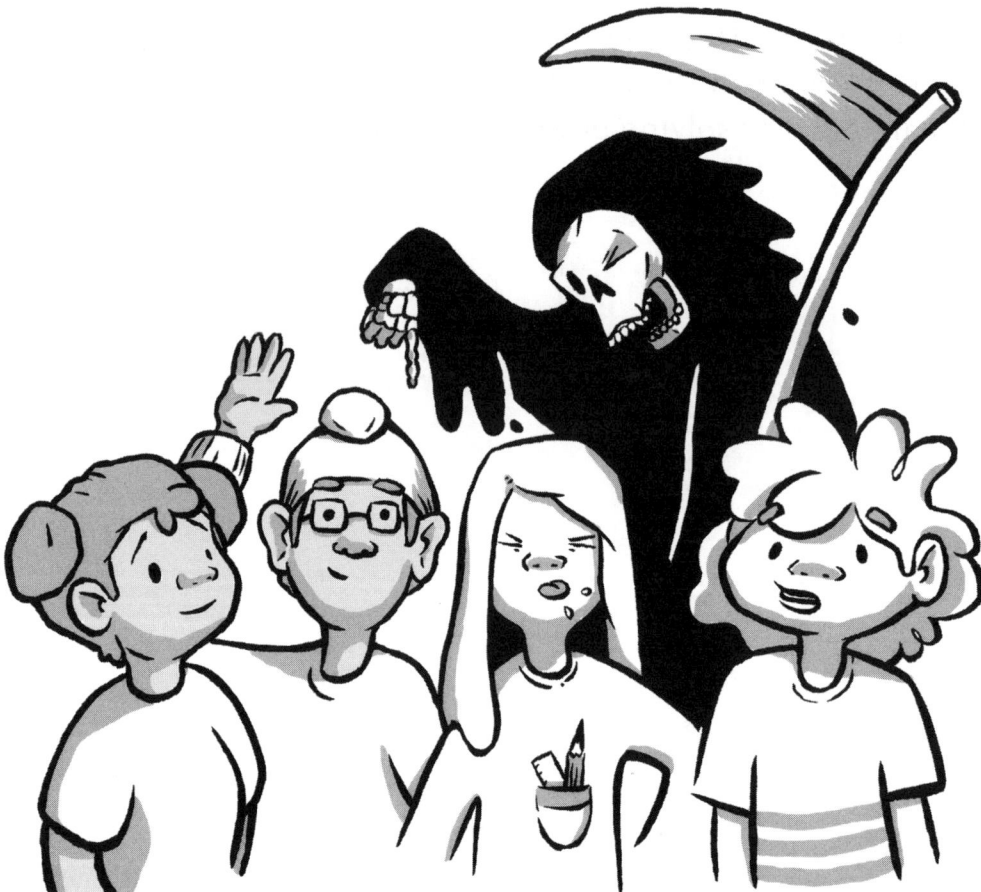

IT solutions

Many of you have already become very good at finding solutions to difficult situations. In the computer screen below, write your favourite computer game. In the outer boxes, write the different things you had to do to reach your goal and become skilled at this game. For example, how did you defeat the dragon? Climb the waterfall? Get through to the next level? You might find it helpful to think of the tips you would give a friend playing the game for the first time.

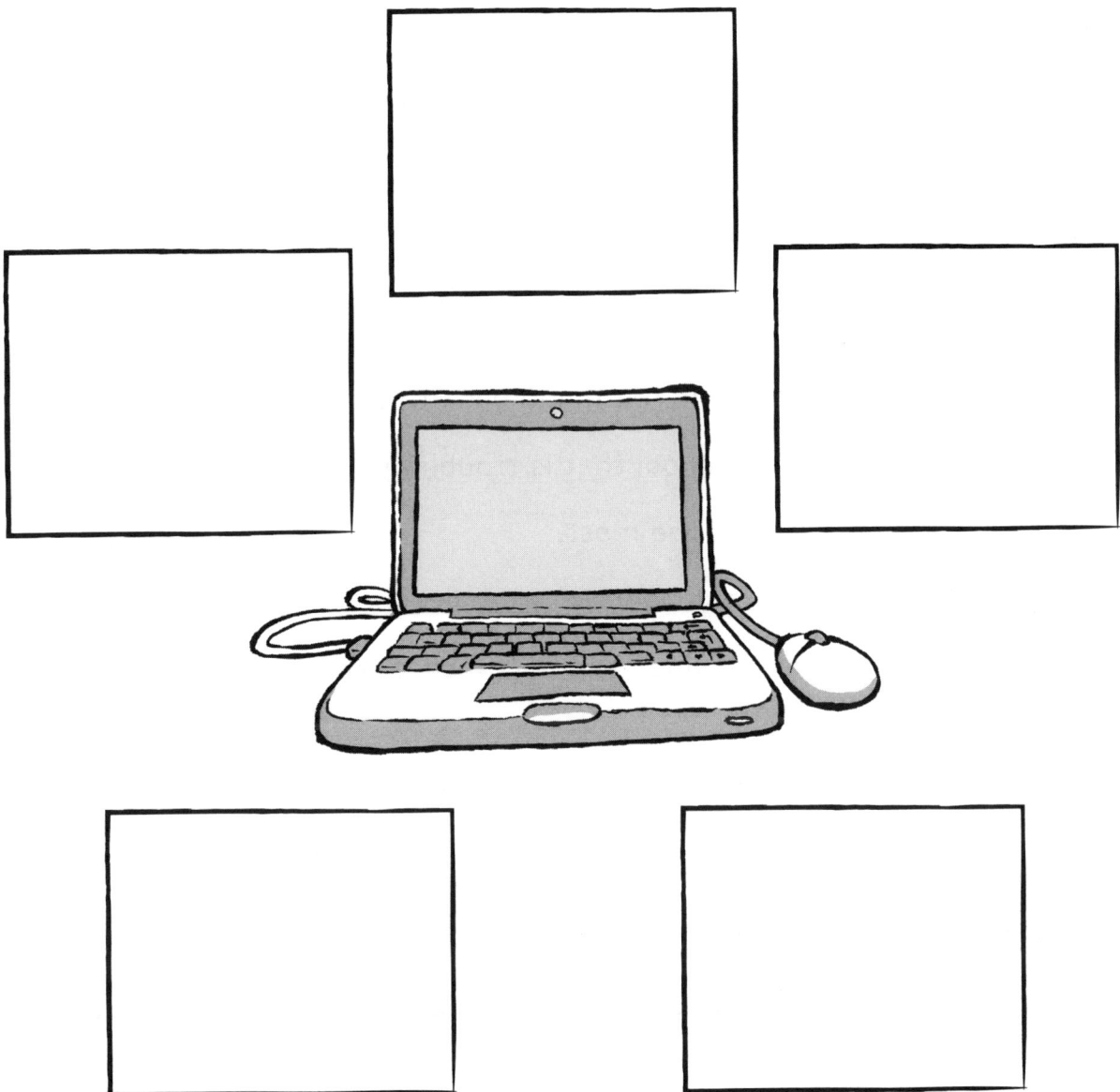

As clear as mud

Many children find it difficult to describe their problems and their goals. They often know something is wrong and they are unhappy but can't explain why. The first cool connection you need to make towards reaching your goal is becoming clear about exactly what is bothering you and where you want to get to. To do this you will need to learn how to be specific and clear like a mountain stream rather than too big and unclear like a muddy river. Make cool connections about which statements are muddy and which are clear from the following examples.

JACK: I hate school and I'm not going back to that dump.

PARENT: What is it about school that is troubling you?

JACK: Everything. I hate everything about school. It's just horrid.

PARENT: Has something happened you are not telling me about?

JACK: No, I just hate school and I'm never ever going back there.

LAUREN: I hate school and I'm not going back to that dump.

PARENT: What is it about school that is troubling you?

LAUREN: I hate break times the most.

PARENT: What is it that is so bad about break times?

LAUREN: Other kids keep calling me a boffin because I'm good at maths and stuff.

PARENT: And what is so bad about being called a boffin?

LAUREN: It makes me feel I'm different like a weird kid or something.

Which child above has most clearly described their problems at school, Jack or Lauren?

If you were a teacher or parent, do you think it would be easier to help Jack or Lauren? Give your reason below.

If you were a teacher or parent trying to help Jack, how would you feel?

From the following problems highlight which are specific and clear and which are too big and muddy.

I'm sure I've got something really wrong with me.

I'm worried because I had a sick feeling in my stomach during games.

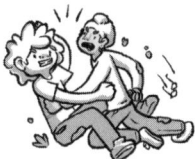

I get bullied all the time by everyone at school.

Amir was hitting me again during first break.

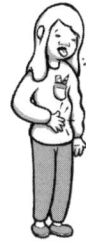

I'm just totally ugly and everyone hates me.

I don't like my hairstyle. It makes me look different from other kids.

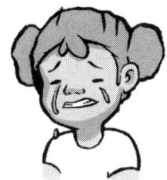

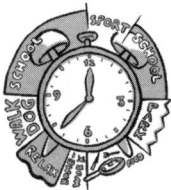

My parents got cross with me this morning because I was late for school again.

Everybody hates me in my family.

I sometimes do well at things.

I got an A Star for my spellings test today in school.

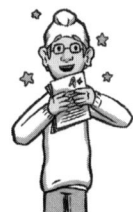

Hoola hoola

Your mission is to solve the following problem by using the A–F goal-setting plan. With the help of a partner, take a hoop and try to get it from one side of the room to the other without touching the hoop with your hands or feet. Think about what you are going to do, and complete the answers to A–D, before you get going with your hoop.

A What is your goal?

. . . .

. . . .

B What could you do to make your goal happen? (ideas)

1. . . . .

2. . . . .

3. . . . .

C What could stop you reaching your goal? (consequences)

1. . . . .

2. . . . .

3. . . . .

D Which of your ideas do you think will work best?

. . . .

. . . .

E Experiment and try out your plan with your partner.

F What happened? Did it work?

Positive outcomes	Things to improve

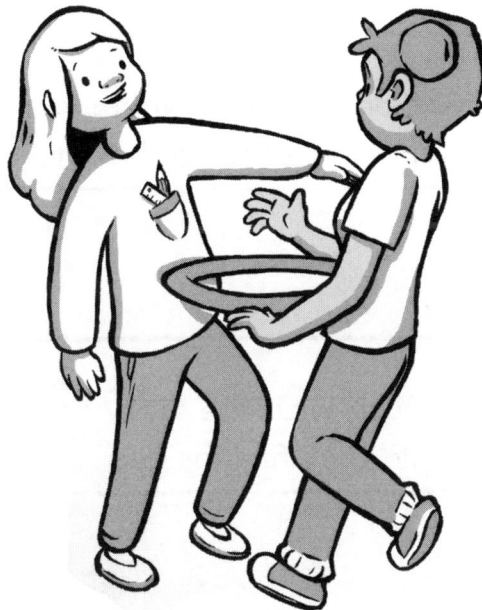

Home activity 9a: Superstars

Sometimes when people get stressed it can be difficult to think of good goal-setting ideas. On these occasions people can feel very stuck. The more stuck they feel, the more stressed they get, like a vicious circle. When you get stuck like this you can get some good ideas for goal setting by thinking about how other people might cope if they were in the same situation. Think of a person you look up to or whom you think copes well in stressful or difficult situations. This could be a superstar from TV, a cartoon character, a family member or even a friend. Complete the information below.

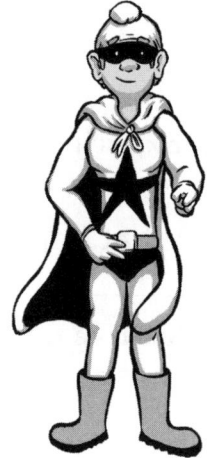

Describe a problem that you think would be very scary or stressful.

Write a goal for making the problem better. (How would you like things to be?)

Write the name of a person or superstar whom you believe would cope well with this situation. (The superstar does not have to be a real person.)

How would your superstar cope with the scary or stressful situation? What would they do and how would they feel inside?

Home activity 9b: Goal setting

Your mission this week is to identify something in your life that is troubling you. Use the A–F goal-setting plan to help you achieve your goal.

A What is your goal?

. . . .

. . . .

B What could you do to make your goal happen (ideas)?

1. . . . .

2. . . . .

3. . . . .

C What could stop you reaching your goal (consequences)?

1. . . . .

2. . . . .

3. . . . .

D Which of your ideas do you think will work best?

. . . .

. . . .

E Experiment and try out your plan with your partner.

F What happened? Did it work?

Positive outcomes	Things to improve

SESSION 10: PANIC CYCLES AND SAFETY-SEEKING ACTIONS

Aims and objectives

- Learn cool connections about how everyone is different and worries about different things.

- See how some of your thoughts and feelings can keep you feeling stuck.

- Find out the different things that people do to protect themselves from their worries and how these can often help feed the problem.

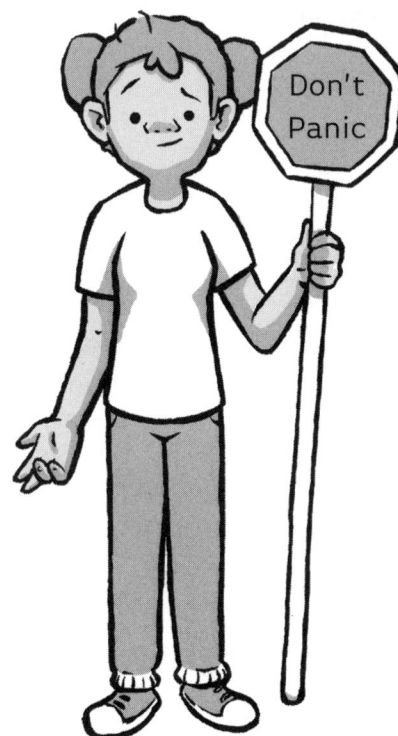

Materials

Chairs, pencils.

Agenda and tips for running the session

Exercises in bold in the left-hand column should be included in both long and short sessions. Other exercises are optional and can be included in groups where there is more time. Many fun activities and games are included as optional. Despite sometimes being short of time it is important not to cut all the 'fun' out of the programme or you will lose the children's enthusiasm.

Short session

EXERCISE	COMMENT
Feedback	Welcome the children and share agenda for session with the group. Obtain brief feedback from the children's week.
Review Home activities 9a and 9b	Children can briefly share one or both home activities. Facilitators collect home activities to explore in more detail after the session and return the following week or at the end of the programme.
The swamp monster	You need a lot of space. Perhaps start the session with this game in a hall or playground. Encourage the children to make the connection between having worries and upset feelings and how these can make you feel very helpless and stuck.
Everyone is different	Some children enjoy reading and can be made to feel more involved. However, this can slow the session down. Children share one or two of the things which they have circled as important to them with the group.
Don't panic!	This exercise helps children to see the links between their thoughts and feelings. Children should be encouraged to notice how worrying thoughts increase physical sensations, forming a vicious cycle.
Put safety first!	Read the story about the children on the train and Jack and his vampires. Many of the children often seem perplexed initially, but eventually most will get the idea. The children can answer the questions either alone or with a partner, and feed back to the group. If you have limited time, read a few of the examples given and ask the children to feed back verbally the safety-seeking actions. Children can then be divided into small groups, given a character from the exercise (Lauren, Katie, Jack or Amir), and asked to either draw, act or identify what they could do differently to overcome their fear.

My safety-seeking actions	If children cannot name something they are afraid of, they can make something up or choose something they know someone else is afraid of.
Home activity 10a: Hidden worries	Children are encouraged to observe their avoidant behaviours.
Home activity 10b: What do I do?	This helps children develop an understanding of their own safety-seeking actions. Children are encouraged to look at how these actions can help or hinder them from coping with their fears.

Long session

Include 'The swamp monster' game. Show an example of safety-seeking actions from a story or online clip. The classic Disney cartoon *Dumbo* is an excellent example. In the film the little elephant Dumbo believes that the only reason he can fly is because he is holding the feather of a bird. It is not until he drops the feather by accident that he suddenly realises that he can fly without it. In the exercises in 'Put safety first!' children can be given more time to choose the characters they would like to act for themselves.

Notes

We have found it useful to suggest that children indicate with a large cross if any of the characters in 'Put safety first!' remind them of themselves. Although most people can identify with all the characters at some point in their lives, children identifying themselves as very similar to the characters (Lauren, Katie, Jack and Amir) on a frequent basis will require further investigation. (These are similar symptoms to those of anxiety disorders such as social phobia, obsessive compulsive disorder or panic attacks.)

The swamp monster

A dangerous and dirty swamp monster has escaped from the depths of a muddy swamp in the land of Piggiwinkles.

If he touches you with his magical muddy fingers you will automatically be stuck like the pig below in a muddy swamp. The only way to be freed from the swamp monster's swampy spell is for another member of your group to crawl through your legs.

If everyone gets swamped by the swamp monster then his powers get stronger and he is the winner.

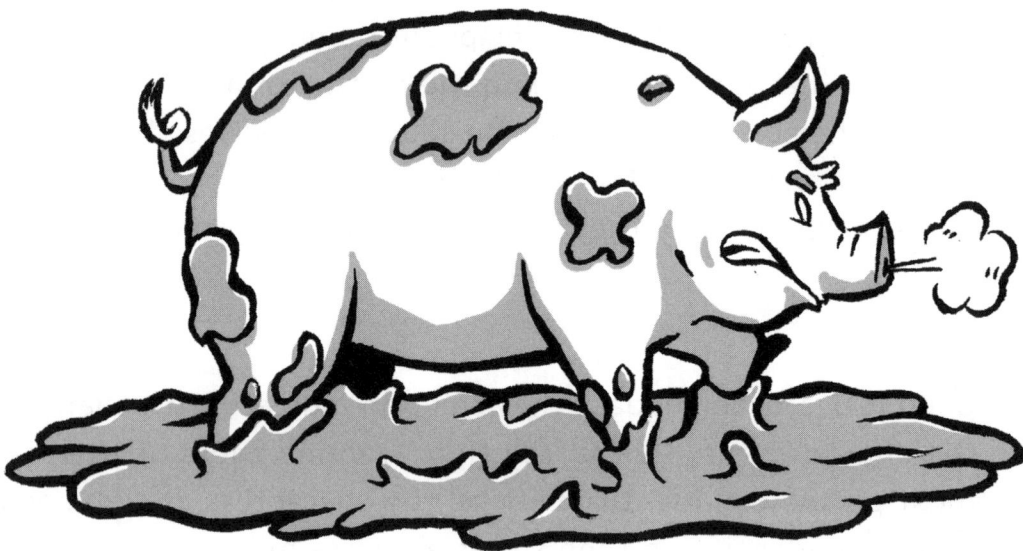

This session helps to show us that:

- sometimes our problems and worries can make us feel very stuck

- sometimes the things we do to help us escape can make us even more stuck

- running away from our fears can make us feel more stuck

- it is good to ask someone to help even if the problem seems too big.

Everyone is different

Everyone is different and will worry about different things. This depends on their values and the things which are important to them. We usually get these values from the experiences we have had in our lives or sometimes from our families. If someone in your family has a strong view about something, you may well share their opinion.

Lauren's mother often tells her that it is wrong to drop litter. Lauren also thinks this is a 'bad' thing to do. However, Jack's mother often throws rubbish out of her car window as she is driving along. Not surprisingly, Jack often drops litter in the street and does not seem bothered about the mess at all. Listed below are some of the things which are important to some children. Circle the things that are important to you.

Being liked by other kids	Being good at sports	Being helpful and kind
Being thin	Being clever at work in school	Being perfect and not making any mistakes
Being tough and hard	Being different from everyone else	Being happy at home and with family
Being caring to animals	Being good at making or fixing things	Being attractive to others

The things you have circled above are very important to you. Because of this you are likely to worry about them. Should something go wrong or you feel you are failing in one of these areas, you are likely to feel very upset. This is sometimes called a trigger. Because we are all different, we all have different triggers for our worries.

Take Fido the dog in the picture below, for example. If someone tried to take his bone he would become very upset and worried. Felix the cat, on the other hand, is not interested in bones, so she wouldn't care who has the bone. However, just you stay away from her cream!

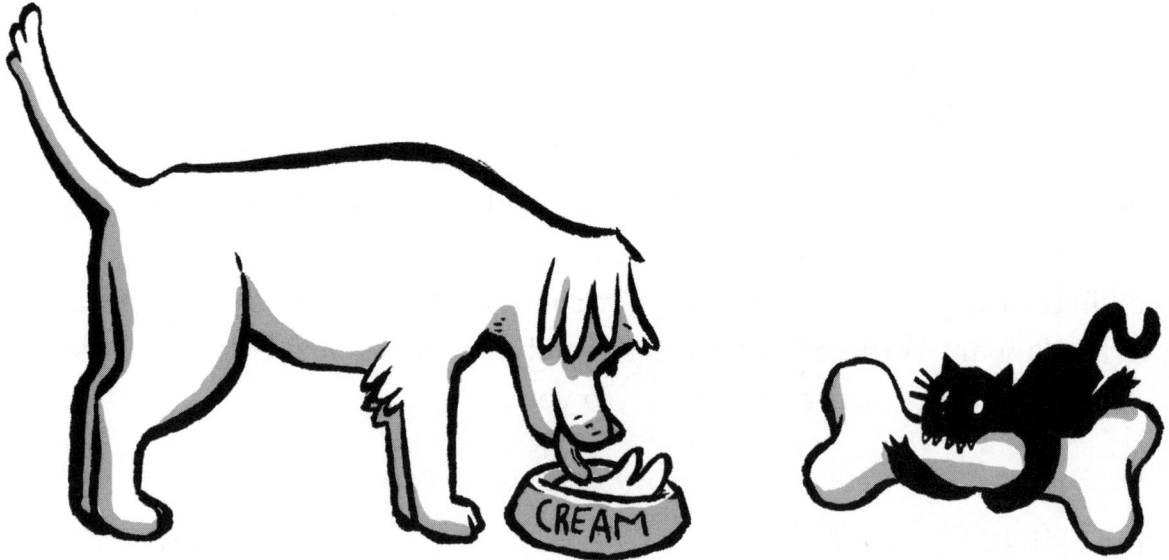

Don't panic!

When people worry, it is always about things in the future and what is going to happen rather than what has happened in the past. It can be very easy to get caught up in a vicious cycle which can make you feel more and more scared and stuck. This cycle is sometimes called the cycle of panic. See the examples of Jack and Katie below:

Jack has been asked to read in front of his class

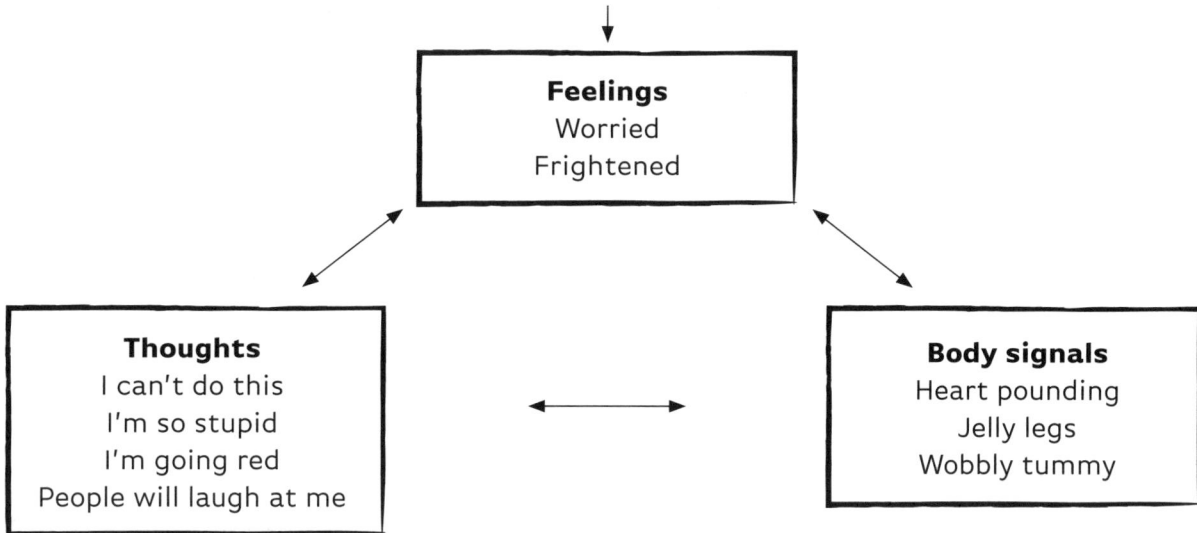

Feelings
Worried
Frightened

Thoughts
I can't do this
I'm so stupid
I'm going red
People will laugh at me

Body signals
Heart pounding
Jelly legs
Wobbly tummy

Some boys laugh at Katie as they walk past

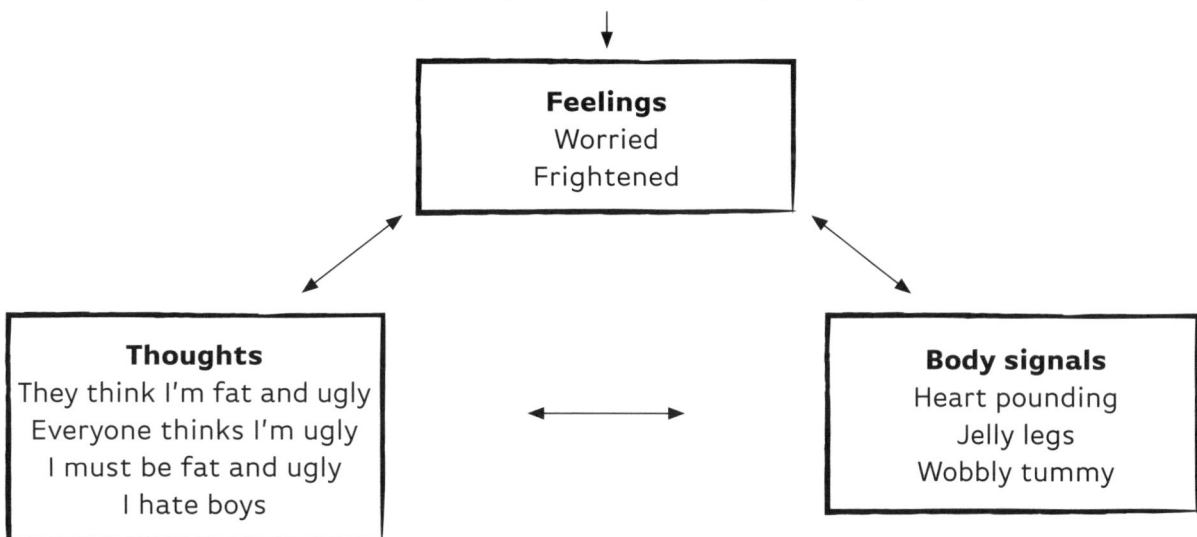

Feelings
Worried
Frightened

Thoughts
They think I'm fat and ugly
Everyone thinks I'm ugly
I must be fat and ugly
I hate boys

Body signals
Heart pounding
Jelly legs
Wobbly tummy

Jack and Katie were bullied during break time.
They fear it could happen again this break time.

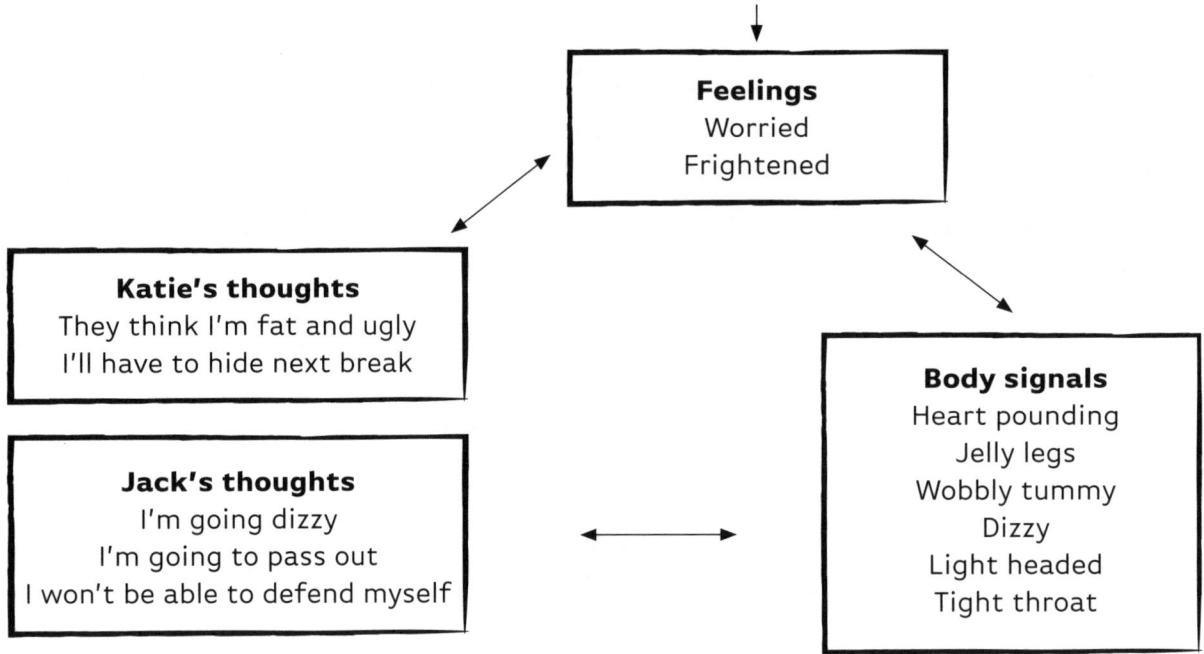

Feelings
Worried
Frightened

Katie's thoughts
They think I'm fat and ugly
I'll have to hide next break

Jack's thoughts
I'm going dizzy
I'm going to pass out
I won't be able to defend myself

Body signals
Heart pounding
Jelly legs
Wobbly tummy
Dizzy
Light headed
Tight throat

Make cool connections by noticing how in different situations both Katie and Jack's worries were different. This is because different things are important to them. Katie seems worried about her good looks and Jack about being physically harmed. Think of a time you have felt worried. In the boxes below see if you can map out your worry cycle.

What happened that made you worried?. . . . .

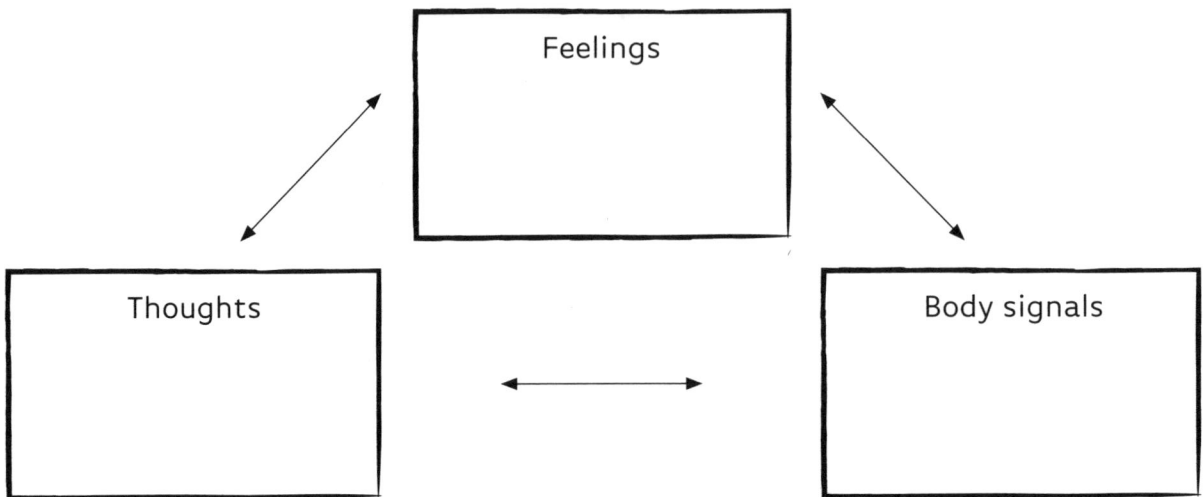

Feelings

Thoughts

Body signals

Put safety first!

Because worrying can be very uncomfortable and causes vicious cycles, people often do things to try and break out. These are called safety-seeking actions. The trouble is that safety-seeking actions often trick you because they seem to help get rid of your worries for a while but then they come back again and can make you feel even more stuck and scared. The following short stories give examples of safety-seeking actions.

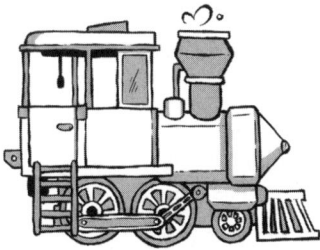

A small group of children are on a train throwing pieces of paper in the air. An older boy calls out, 'What are you doing?' They reply, 'Keeping elephants out of the train.' The older boy looks surprised and shouts back, 'But there are no elephants in this country and certainly not on this train.' 'Yes,' said the children playfully. 'Our strategy works really well doesn't it!'

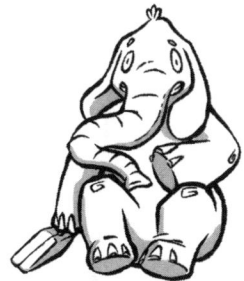

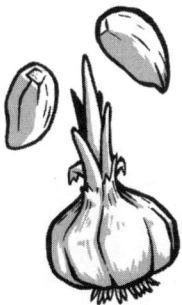

Jack invites his three friends – Amir, Katie and Lauren – to his house for a special party tea which he has cooked himself. When they arrive, they notice lots of garlic hanging from the doorway and neatly placed across the windowsill in the kitchen. 'Strange,' they think, but they don't like to ask. 'Perhaps they are for the party?' Jack proudly presents the first course, which is garlic bread. Very tasty too! For the main course, Jack has made garlic chicken, which arrives on a tray with rather odd-tasting drinks in garlic-shaped glasses. Finally, for pudding, his friends laugh when he produces a special type of garlic ice cream. Jack seems puzzled as to why his guests are laughing, so eventually Lauren asks, 'What is it with all the garlic?' Jack is silent for a minute, then he says in a very serious tone, 'It's to keep the vampires away of course.' Amir, Katie and Lauren laugh again before Amir says, 'But there are no vampires.' 'Exactly,' says Jack, smiling to himself. 'The garlic has kept them away.'

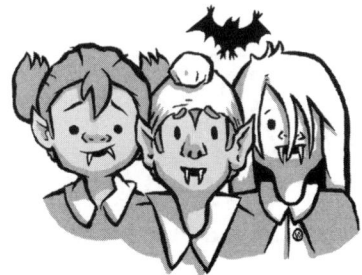

Why does Jack keep so much garlic in his house?

What safety-seeking actions does Jack do to keep himself safe?

Do you think Jack's idea about keeping so much garlic is helping him overcome his fear of vampires? If so, how?

What would have to happen for Jack to find out the vampires do not exist? How would you advise him?

With a partner, make cool connections by seeing how many safety-seeking actions you can detect from the characters below and circle each one. Choose one character and show (by acting, writing or drawing) what they could do differently to help them cope with or overcome their fear.

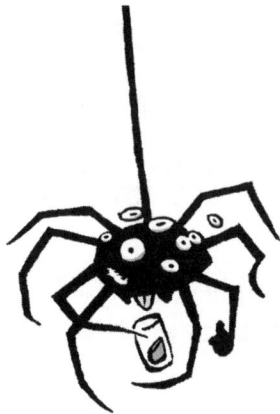

Lauren is scared of spiders. Each time she sees one she starts to feel panicky and runs away as fast as she can. Although she feels better when she gets away from the spider, she feels really silly next time she sees her friends. She spends a lot of time looking for spiders and won't go into a room if she so much as sees something that looks like a spider. She spends more time looking for spiders than doing her lessons.

Katie is worried about what people think of her, so she spends hours practising what she says to people in her mirror at home just in case she says the wrong thing. Unless she has practised what to say, she does not speak most of the time just in case she upsets someone.

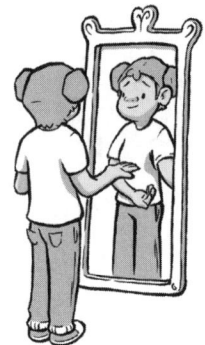

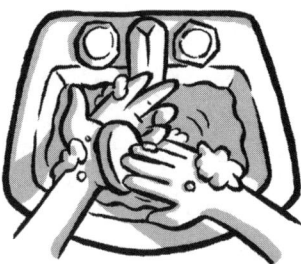

Jack is worried about catching germs, so he washes his hands over and over again to prevent getting germs and being ill. If he doesn't wash his hands in a certain order he feels he must start washing them all over again. With all this washing, his hands have become quite sore.

Amir's dad died of a heart attack. Sometimes when he gets panicky his chest gets tight and he thinks he will pass out and have a heart attack too. Even though the doctor has said there is nothing wrong with him, he always holds on to something to stop himself falling if he feels worried. Just in case!

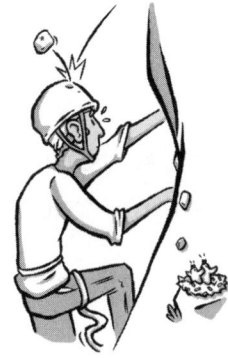

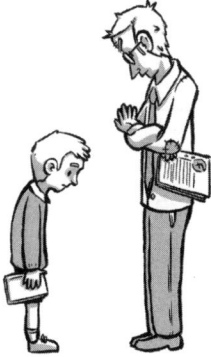

Jack does not like school because he keeps getting into trouble. He gets really panicky just thinking about school. He tells his mum that he has got a headache or feels sick. She lets him stay at home because she is so worried. Jack gets bored at home but he won't go back, just in case the horrid feelings of worry come back too.

Lauren plays tennis in a top club. She is very good and has never lost a match. The first time she played in a tennis match, someone told her that she would play well if she spins her racket ten times before each service. She is fed up with doing this now but is worried that if she stops she will lose the match.

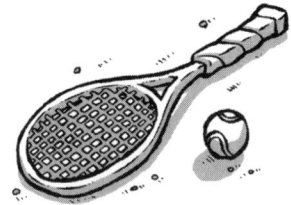

My safety-seeking actions

Name something that you are afraid of (e.g. spiders, heights, parents arguing, blushing in public, etc.).

What things do you do to avoid facing your fear or stop it happening (e.g. washing your hands to avoid germs, not going near spiders, thinking about something else)?

What would be the worst thing that would happen if you came face to face with your fear but could not escape or do the things above (e.g. pass out, die, go crazy, scream and shout, get laughed at)?

Home activity 10a: Hidden worries

Many people find it difficult to think of things that they are afraid of. That's because we usually don't admit to ourselves that we're scared. We say 'I know my limits' and 'I don't see the point', or 'I don't want to' and 'Why should I?' We stop doing things that make us feel scared, because feeling scared is uncomfortable. Make cool connections by looking at things you avoid doing and ask yourself, 'Is it actually because I'm afraid?' Here are some examples:

KATIE: 'I don't want to go to the party. It's not cool' (I'm also scared of being laughed at because I can't find any nice clothes to wear. They all make me look fat and ugly).

AMIR: 'I don't want to play football on the field today – it's boring' (actually I'm frightened there may be a snake lurking in the long grass).

LAUREN: 'I don't want to play in the tennis match – I'm too tired' (and also I'm scared I will let my partner and the team down if I don't play well).

JACK: 'It's too late for you to come to my house for supper' (I'm also scared my parents will be arguing again and that would be embarrassing).[1]

Write some things you don't like doing in the box below. Circle the things you avoid doing because of fear.

---

1   Adapted from Alexander, J. (2006) *Bullies, Bigmouths and So-Called Friends*. London: Hodder Children's Books. Text copyright Jenny Alexander 2003. Reproduced and adapted by permission of Hodder and Stoughton Limited.

Home activity 10b: What do I do?

Think of a time that you felt really afraid, worried or panicky. Complete the lines and boxes below.

What happened? . . . .

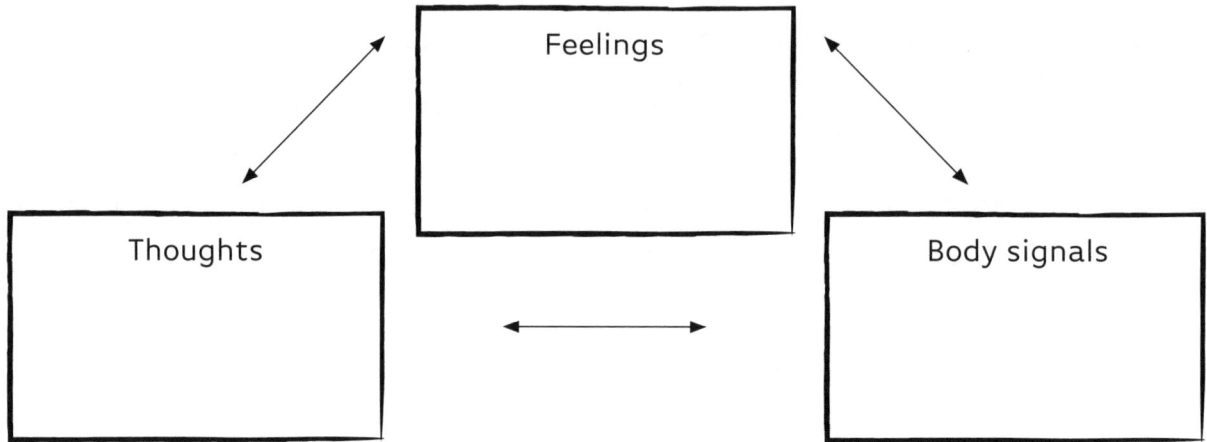

. . . .

```
        Feelings

Thoughts          Body signals
```

List the things that you did (safety-seeking actions) to reduce your worries and calm yourself down – for example, run away, stay at home.

1. . . . .

2. . . . .

3. . . . .

If there is anything you could do differently to help you face your fear next time, write it in the box below.

SESSION 11: FACING YOUR FEARS

Aims and objectives

- Learn how to break your problems into smaller, more achievable steps.

- Show how imagining yourself achieving your goals can be helpful.

- Show how modelling yourself on someone who copes well can help you overcome your fears.

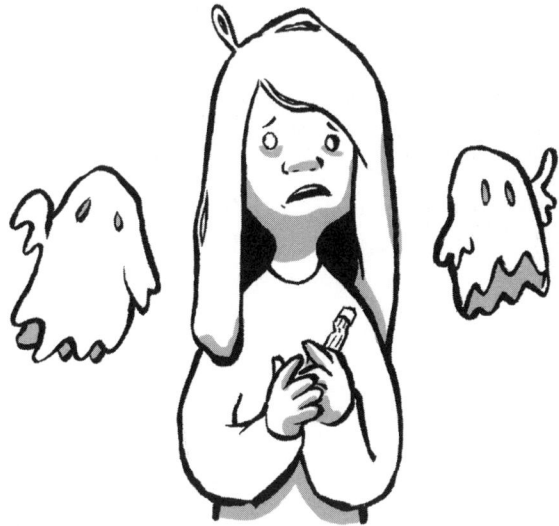

Materials

Chairs, pencils, shoe with a lace.

Agenda and tips for running the session

Exercises in bold in the left-hand column should be included in both long and short sessions. Other exercises are optional and can be included in groups where there is more time. Many fun activities and games are included as optional. Despite sometimes being short of time it is important not to cut all the 'fun' out of the programme or you will lose the children's enthusiasm.

Short session

EXERCISE	COMMENT
Feedback	Welcome the children and share agenda for session with the group. Obtain brief feedback from the children's week.
Review Home activities 10a and 10b	Children can briefly discuss their home activities. Facilitators collect home activities to explore in more detail after the session and return the following week or at the end of the programme.
One two I can lace my shoe	Give children two minutes to complete the exercise. Compare the number of steps children have identified. Choose a volunteer to pretend to be an alien and see if he or she can carry out the steps. Unless the steps are broken down clearly, it is unlikely that the instructions can be followed.
Feel the fear	Read the anecdote to the children and conduct the 'pink elephants theory' in the session. This exercise will illustrate that the harder you avoid or push away 'scary thoughts' the more frightening they become and the more difficult they are to overcome. This exercise is also closely linked with the safety-seeking actions described in Session 10.
Cutting your fear down	This illustrates how a fear can develop and be overcome. Children can be asked to volunteer their own experiences of overcoming fears. How did they do it? Who helped them? How do they feel about the fear now?
Step by step	Read through the steps Miss Muffet took to overcome her fear of spiders.

My step plan	Children are encouraged to be specific about what they want to achieve (their goal) and write this at the top of their step plan (step 7). Having identified this goal they can either start at step 1 and work up in small steps or work backwards from their goal at step 7. Children are then encouraged to share their step plans with the group. If children cannot identify a specific fear they can make up a step plan that would help a friend or relative. Learning the process is the important thing in this exercise. If they understand the basic concepts then they can apply the principles to their own fears and difficulties when they are ready.
Home activity 11a: Imagine, imagine, imagine	The exercise is aimed at helping children visualise themselves coming to terms with their fears. Many people are so avoidant of their fears that simply imagining the fear is a huge step towards coping. For children to visualise themselves just being with their fear can be very empowering and can help boost their confidence.
Home activity 11b: How we face our fears	This encourages children to work together to generate new ways of coping.

Long session

Include 'One two I can lace my shoe'. Children can be asked to write a short story or draw a picture about a fear. They can create a character and write/draw about how they overcame the fear using some of the skills they have learned (green-light thoughts, visualising themselves coping, breaking the fear into small steps, etc.). Alternatively, children can act out their step plans with a partner and show them to the rest of the group.

One two I can lace my shoe

Imagine you have met an alien. He wants you to teach him how to tie his shoe laces. As the alien has never worn shoes before and he does not understand things like 'make a bow' or 'just thread it through there', you are going to have to break your instructions into very small steps and be very clear so that he can understand. List your instructions in the table below. See who in your group can list the most number of steps.

Give your list to a friend and see if they can follow the steps if they do exactly what your instructions say.

Lace my shoe: instructions for an alien

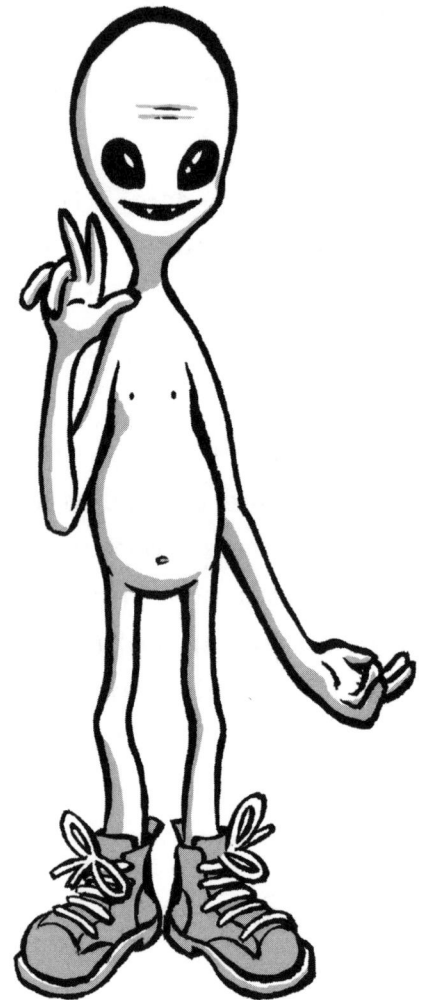

Feel the fear and do it anyway

Most people who have a fear or worry try to avoid it at all costs. They don't want to hear about it, think about it or talk about it, and most of all they don't want to have to face it. They just want it to go away. The trouble is that worries don't always just go away. In fact, sometimes the more you try to avoid or not think about your worries, the more they seem to bug you.

Pink elephants theory

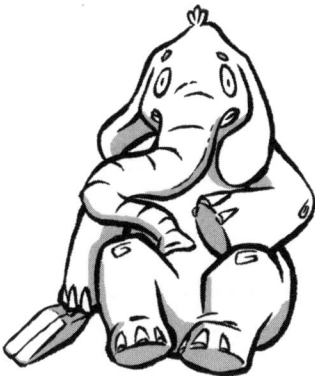

As an example of this, close your eyes and try really hard not to think about pink elephants. What happened? Most people find that they think about pink elephants. This goes to show that the more you try not to think about something the worse it becomes.

The truth is that the only real way to completely get rid of your worries is to face up to them. Like the saying goes, 'Feel the fear and do it anyway'.

This is easier said than done, but some ideas that might help you include:

- Thinking green-light thoughts (see Session 8).

- Take small steps.

- Imagine yourself achieving your goals or coping with your problem or fear.

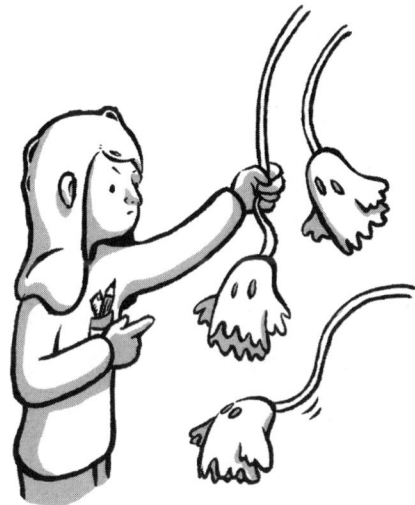

Cutting your fears down

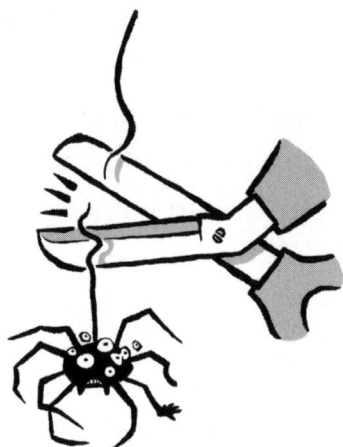

Everyone knows that if you fall off a horse you should get back in the saddle as soon as possible. That's because when you've had a bad experience you fear it could happen again, and the sooner you face up to the fear, the easier it is to get over it. The longer you put off facing up to fear, the bigger it grows. By the time the fear's got bigger than you, there's no way you can tackle it head on. You have to work up to it in stages, starting with smaller fears first.

Lauren's high dive

Lauren has been having diving coaching at the local swimming pool. She really enjoys it and is doing well. She can do lots of different dives. She can go backwards and she can even do a somersault into the water. The trouble is that since she did a belly flop a few years ago, she has become too afraid to dive from the top board. Her parents have offered her a present if she can pluck up the courage, but it just seems too high. When Lauren looks down from the edge of the high board, her legs feel like jelly and her knees knock together. She thinks to herself, 'It's just too scary. I'm sure to hurt myself.' Frightening pictures flash through her head of belly flops, people laughing at her, and hospitals. Poor Lauren believes that she will never learn to dive from the top board.

Lauren's coach does not despair. He patiently encourages her to practise an easy dive over and over again from the side of the swimming pool. Gradually she progresses from the poolside on to the first board. Lauren uses a step-by-step approach to face her fear. Once Lauren has perfected the first diving board, her coach encourages her to go higher and dive from the second board. Although she is a little nervous to begin with, she quickly gains confidence and dives beautifully. She even completes a few somersaults to show off her skills to her mum and dad who are watching in the swimming pool gallery.

Eventually Lauren's coach suggests she try from the top. Nervously, Lauren stands on the end of the board. It does not seem so high this time, after all her practice. Having pictured herself doing the dive successfully in her mind as her coach instructed, Lauren raises her arms, then pauses for a moment before jumping high into the air. She feels the wind rush through her hair and her body whizz round as she completes the dive and plunges through the water perfectly. Success. She has done it. Her parents and coach clap as she rushes up the steps of the diving board with excitement to do it all over again. Lauren has taken small steps and overcome her fear.

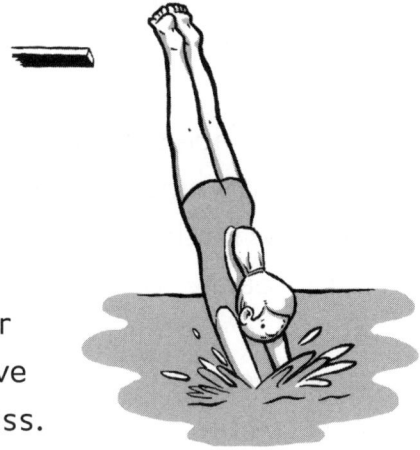

Can you think of a time when you overcame a fear like Lauren in the example above? How did you cut your fear down to size?

Step by step

In order to face something that you are afraid of, it can be helpful to break the fear into small steps. In the example below, make cool connections by seeing how Little Miss Muffet overcomes her fear of spiders using a step-by-step approach. You do not have to be afraid of spiders to use this approach. In fact, this same approach can be used to overcome any fear from heights, water, insects, mice, talking in public, sickness or school. The most important thing is to start with your goal in step 7. This should contain what you want to be able to do when you have overcome your fear. Note that Little Miss Muffet does not have to like spiders to get over her fear. She is satisfied just to have one walk on her hand.

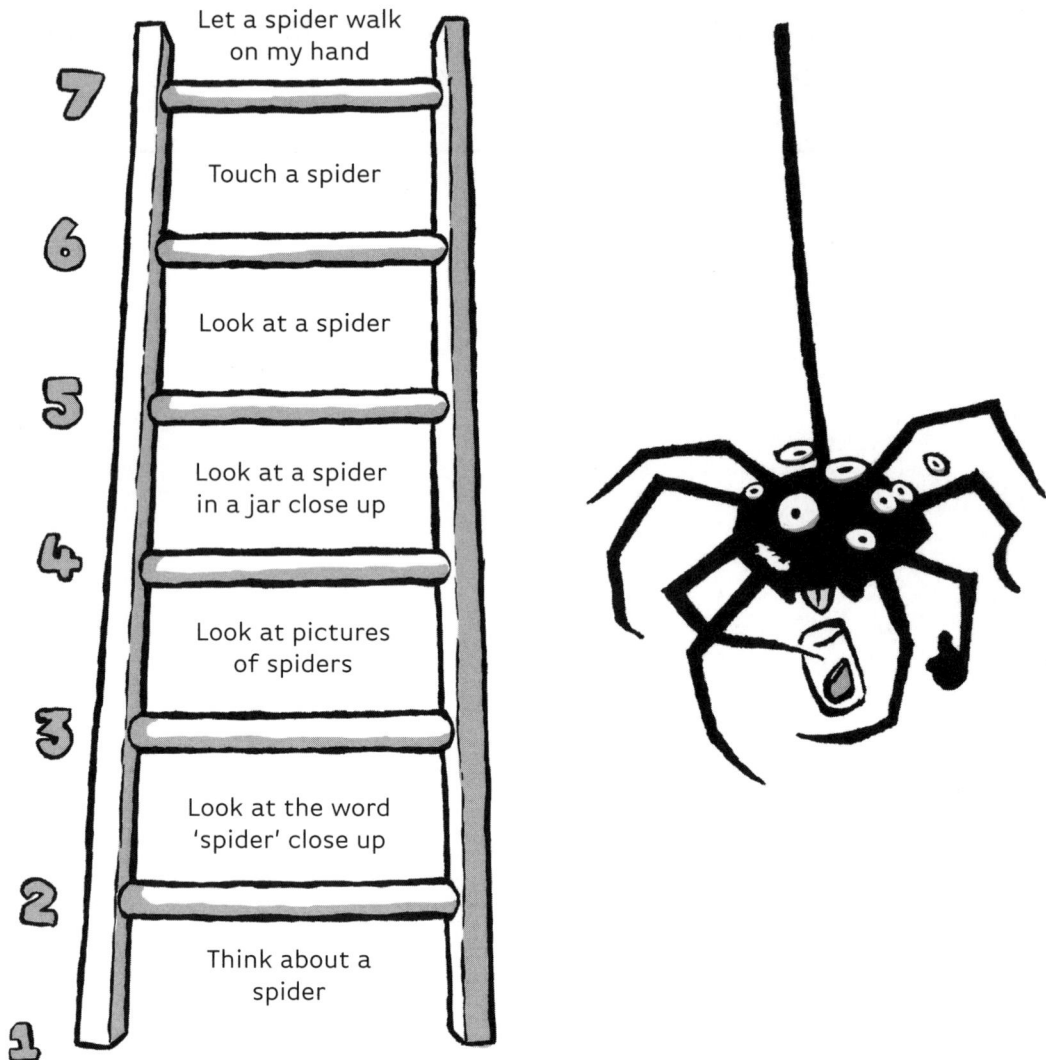

7 — Let a spider walk on my hand

6 — Touch a spider

5 — Look at a spider

4 — Look at a spider in a jar close up

3 — Look at pictures of spiders

2 — Look at the word 'spider' close up

1 — Think about a spider

My step plan

As no two people are the same, everyone's step-by-step ladder will be different. To begin, write your goal at the top of your ladder (step 7). Following this, complete steps 1 to 6, with step 1 as the easiest step and the rest getting more difficult. The smaller the steps the more likely you are to achieve your goal.

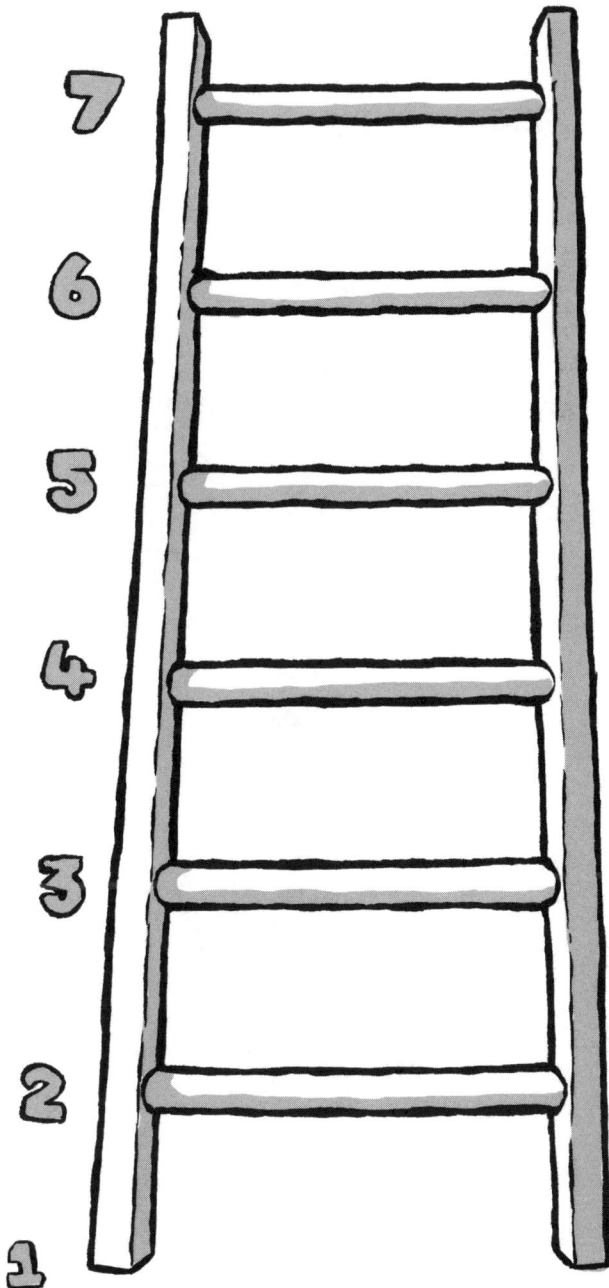

Home activity 11a: Imagine, imagine, imagine

To overcome problems or fears it can be very helpful to imagine yourself coping. Let your mind go wild and dream up some cool ways to overcome your fears. Use magic to turn the bullies into frogs, dive from the top diving board, get an A in your science test or imagine super powers to cope with frightening monsters. Whatever, make sure you come out on top. Either draw or use modelling materials to create your scene. Share your ideas with the group.

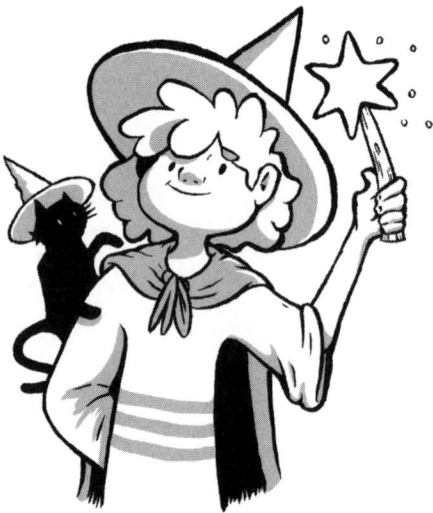

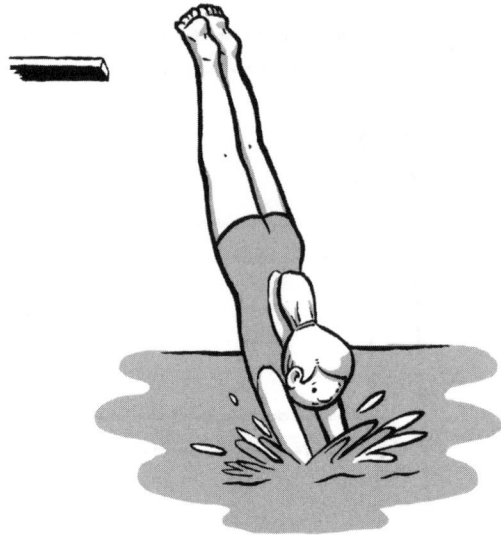

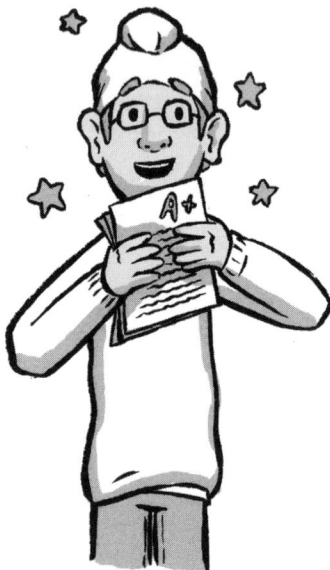

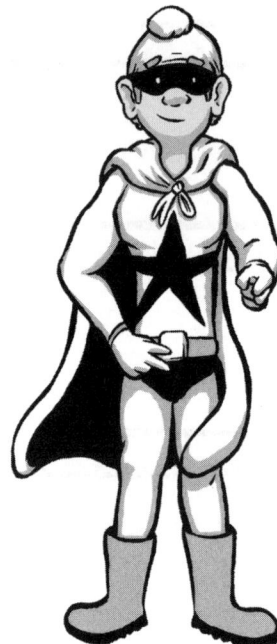

Home activity 11b: How we face our fears

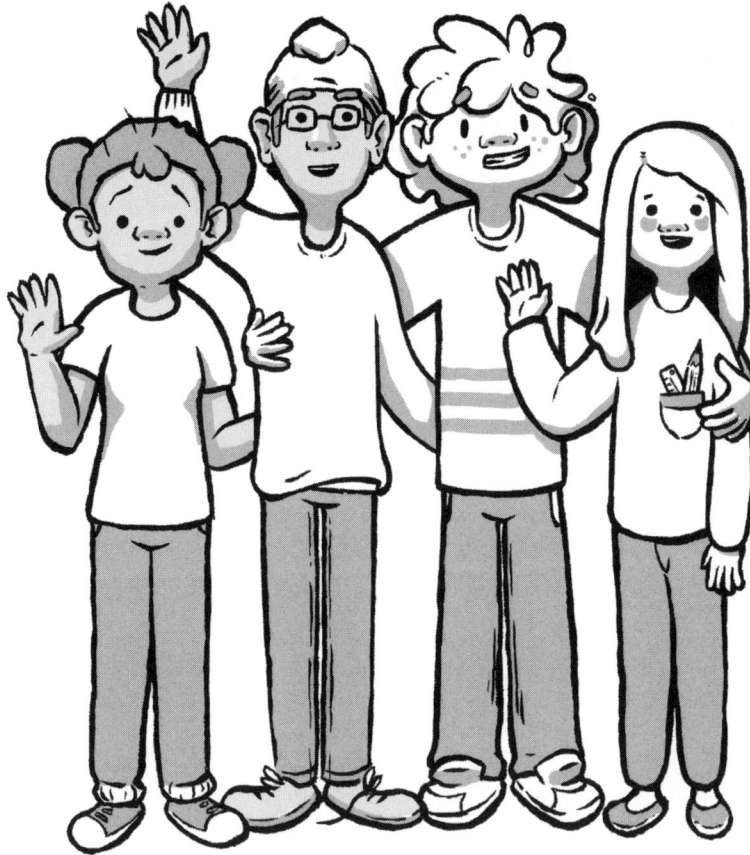

Get together with a friend from the group during the week. Design a poster, or make a little show, dance or pop song, to demonstrate how you made cool connections to face your fears. Performances will take place next session and should last no longer than three minutes each. Try to include as many of the following ways of coping in your presentation:

- Taking small steps

- Imagine yourself coping

- Thinking of how a good 'coper' could tackle your fears

- Thinking green-light thoughts.

SESSION 12: MINDFULNESS

Aims and objectives

- Learn about mindfulness and the benefits of being in the 'present moment'.

- Become kinder and less judgemental about ourselves.

- Develop an awareness of both inner and outer experiences.

- Recognise your thoughts as 'just thoughts'.

- Be grateful and focus on the things we have rather than the things which we have not.

Materials

Pens or pencils. Chocolate or alternative healthy food if running the longer session.

Agenda and tips for running the session

Exercises in bold in the left-hand column should be included in both long and short sessions. To save time in shorter sessions, omit 'Mindful chocolate eating' and/or 'Leaves on a stream visualisation'. This is at the discretion of the facilitator.

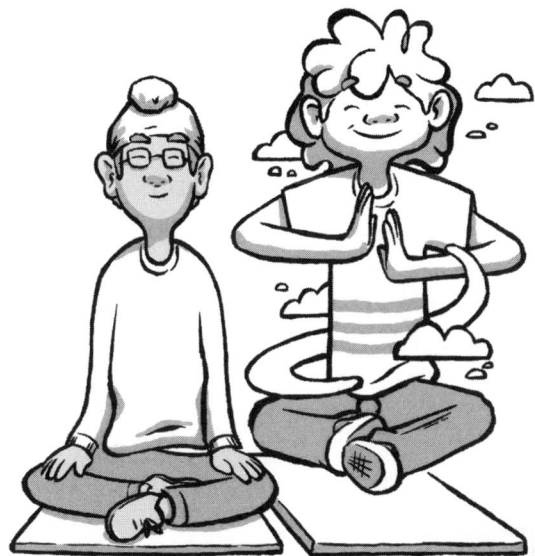

Short session

EXERCISE	COMMENT
Welcome children	Share agenda for Session 12 with the group.
Review Home activities 11a and 11b	Group members briefly show how they completed homework tasks and share with the rest of the group. Note any observations made by children. What ideas did they generate? How did using their imagination help?
A way for the worrier	The group are encouraged to read about how the act of mindfulness is an ancient tradition and an art form – something that requires practice rather than just a technique in a book. It may be useful for individuals to identify times when or activities in which they have acted mindfully.
Mindful breathing exercise	In Session 4, the group experimented with relaxation and hyperventilation, learning about how this affects our physiology. This exercise is more about awareness. The facilitator reads aloud the 'Breathe in, breathe out' exercise and the group are encouraged to focus all of their attention on their breathing. This is a first step in helping individuals be in the 'present moment'. It may be useful to point out how difficult this is to do as children's minds are frequently thinking about school, friends, hobbies and more. Children are invited to fully experience being present in each moment.
Mindful chocolate eating	Although this exercise involves chocolate, some facilitators may prefer to use healthier foods. Raisins, for example, are often used in teaching mindfulness. The point is for group members to experience eating something mindfully and to notice how this is different from their normal experience of eating. Some children may comment that the food tastes better, or how they usually eat too fast or in front of the television and miss out on the flavour. Children may also notice that a lack of awareness may cause some people to eat too much.

Gratitude

This is a topic which many parents and teachers may notice young people often lack. However, the purpose of gratitude relating to mindfulness is not only to show gratitude towards others but also to one's self. Many individuals are kind and have gratitude towards others, but are quite mean towards themselves. This can lead to anxiety, low mood and issues with self-esteem. Learning to have gratitude towards ourselves helps validate our feelings. Group members can learn that this strategy in itself is a powerful tool in relieving stress and staying cool.

Mindfulness of thoughts and feelings

Encourage the group to read through the information about thoughts. It can be very enlightening for some children to realise that their thoughts are 'normal' and everyone has 'bad or uncomfortable' thoughts sometimes. Angry thoughts or thoughts of wanting to harm someone can be very scary. Consequently, many children will keep them as a secret. It is important to distinguish between individuals who want to carry out harmful thoughts and children who have occasional bad thoughts that make them feel upset. While it is quite normal to think angry or aggressive thoughts sometimes, facilitators should seek medical advice if any group members have frequent thoughts about harming themselves or other people – especially so if they report making plans to act out these thoughts (see also section below – 'It's what you do and say that counts'). As described in 'Confidentiality' (in the Group Facilitators' Guide) at the beginning of this programme, any facilitator who considers a child could be at risk needs to follow the safeguarding procedure in their workplace, or discuss with a qualified professional such as social services or possibly their GP.

It's what you do and say that counts

This highlights that everyone has different thoughts. It is useful to notice our thoughts and how they come and go, perhaps like advertisements behind aeroplanes or leaves on a stream. There is a link between thoughts, feelings and what we do. Awareness of our thoughts gives us more choices.

Leaves on a stream visualisation	This is a mindfulness exercise to help group members to just notice their thoughts. If children suggest they haven't got any thoughts ('my mind has gone blank'), encourage them to put that thought or the fact that their mind has gone blank on to a leaf to flow downstream. The group can be reminded that images or feelings can also float down the stream.
Light stream visualisation	Many people avoid uncomfortable feelings. This exercise illustrates how when we accept and move closer to our feelings they are more likely to get processed and float away. As described above, when we avoid or try to work out our feelings, they tend to intensify and become more uncomfortable. Frequently when children find this exercise difficult, it is because they are not truly willing to accept their feelings. If children find this exercise difficult, just help them notice that it is difficult and move on.
Mindfulness overview	This provides four elements which are mindfulness strategies to help children calm themselves down. Practising the four elements regularly will help improve children's personal resilience and ability to self-soothe.
Home activity 12: Mindfulness	As already suggested, mindfulness takes practice. Facilitators should encourage the group to keep note of things they do mindfully this week. This can be anything from cleaning their teeth and walking to school, to eating lunch.

Long session

More time can be spent discussing each exercise with the group. Facilitators could also show pictures or a YouTube clip of leaves floating on a stream. Also include 'Mindful chocolate eating' and/or 'Leaves on a stream visualisation'. There are a number of mindfulness exercises that can be found online (such as GoZen! Mindfulness Exercises for Kids) which can be watched as a practice exercise or to enhance understanding.

Notes

The exercises in this session are aimed at teaching mindfulness skills. This also helps build self-awareness and personal resilience. Mindfulness skills are thought to help reduce stress and anxiety, strengthen attention and focus, support social and emotional growth, and better resolve the inevitable conflicts that arise in children's lives.

A way for the worrier

Mindfulness is very old and is often linked with Eastern meditation, including yoga, and some martial arts such as the ancient art of the Samurai Sword. Mindfulness skills can take a lifetime to learn. For that reason, some aspects of mindfulness are sometimes considered as 'The way of the warrior'. In this session, you will learn how this mystic art can help you calm your body and mind. With practice, you will cope better with your emotions and feel happier in yourself. Mindfulness is about *noticing what is happening right now, in the present moment and without judgement.* This means noticing what is happening around you and the cool connections between your body and mind.

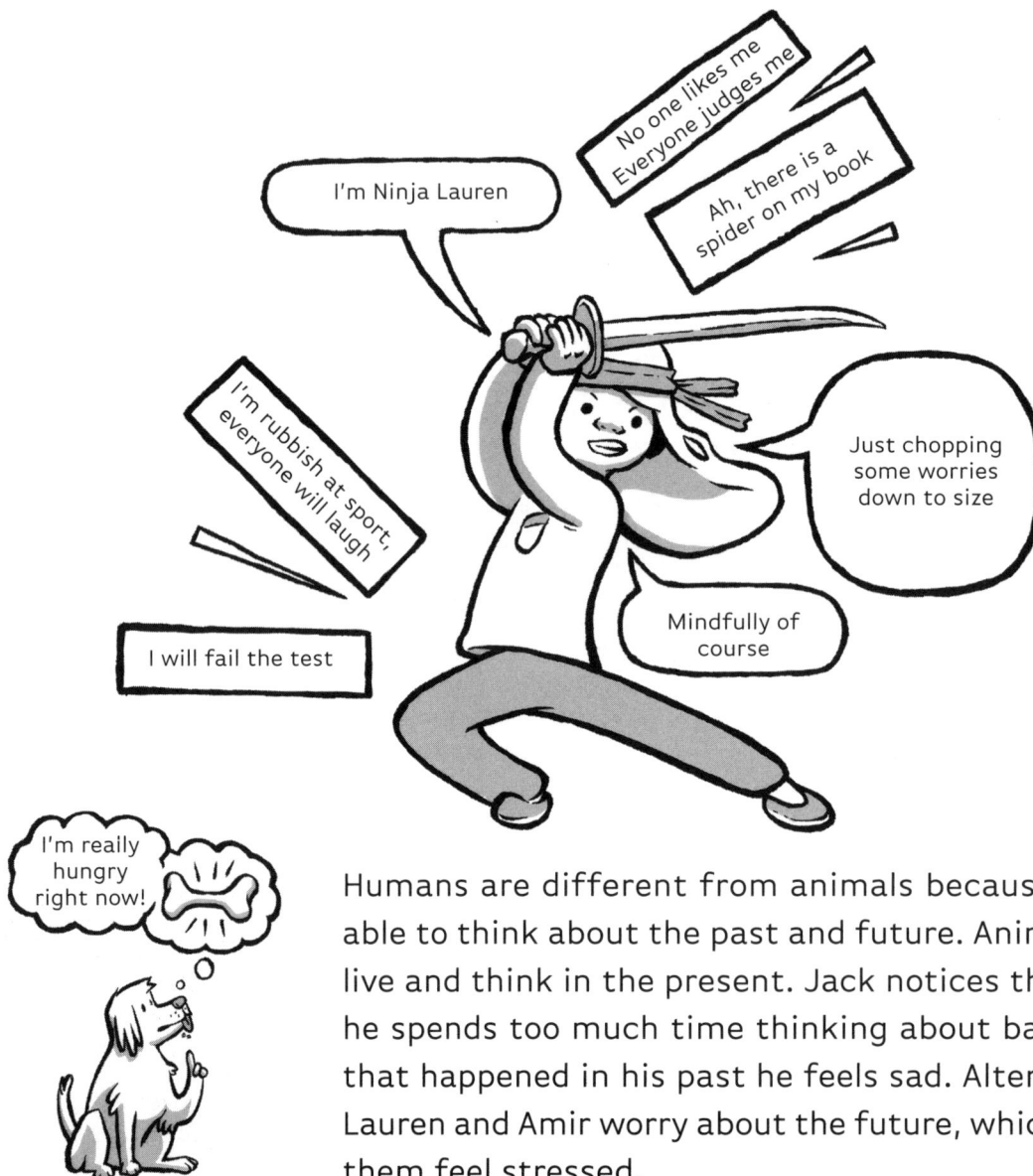

No one likes me Everyone judges me

Ah, there is a spider on my book

I'm Ninja Lauren

I'm rubbish at sport, everyone will laugh

Just chopping some worries down to size

Mindfully of course

I will fail the test

I'm really hungry right now!

Humans are different from animals because we are able to think about the past and future. Animals only live and think in the present. Jack notices that when he spends too much time thinking about bad things that happened in his past he feels sad. Alternatively, Lauren and Amir worry about the future, which makes them feel stressed.

We are often so lost in the past or in the future we miss out on what is going on in the present. Look around at home or school and you may notice lots of people seem lost in their thoughts. Even when listening or speaking to someone in the present, we are not always 'present'. This sometimes gets Jack and Katie into trouble.

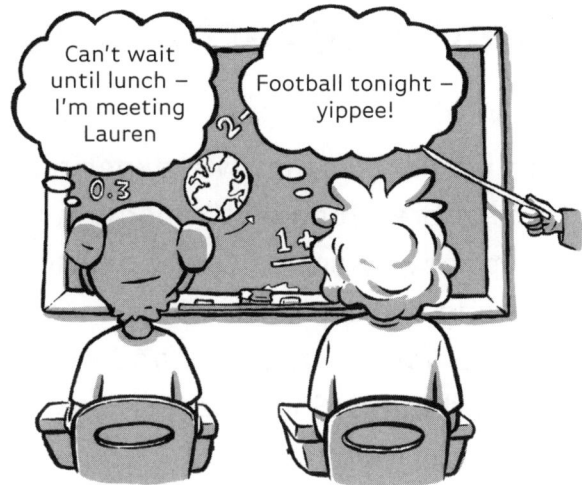

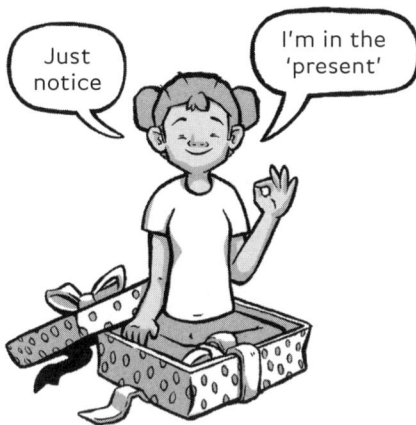

Mindfulness helps break this trap. It also helps us feel calmer, focused and more present in the moment. Frequently people spend too much time daydreaming without being aware of what is going on 'in the here and now'. It's as if we're trapped inside our minds. As a wise ninja once said: 'Yesterday is history. Tomorrow a mystery. Today is a gift and that's why it is called the "present".'

There is a book called *You Are Special* by Max Lucado, about wooden people who give each other stars and dots. The characters notice that the stars and dots do not stick to people who trust their own judgement and do not believe the negative comments made by the other wooden people. This is like the 'non-judgement' part of mindfulness. Just notice – without judgement. Some children are very good at judging other people, but these individuals are rarely 'mindful' about themselves or how their comments affect others.

We have already learned that the way we think affects the way we feel and what we do. In this session, we are learning to be more mindful and in the 'present moment'. With this new awareness, we hope to become more compassionate and less judgemental of ourselves and other people.

Mindful breathing exercise

In an earlier session, we experimented with the effect of breathing on the body. In this exercise, we learn to pay attention to the physical sensations of breathing and explore a mindfulness technique that can help you to stay cool and feel calmer in your body and mind. Some people describe themselves as having 'monkey minds'. This is because their thoughts are like monkeys jumping about all over the place and having difficulty relaxing, focusing or staying calm.

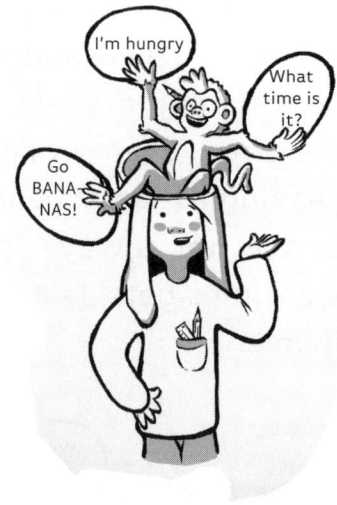

The following exercise is a grounding exercise which can help you in the present moment and to gain some control if you have trouble with a 'monkey mind' – especially if your mind wants to get up to 'monkey business' and won't keep still or quiet.

Breathe in, breathe out...

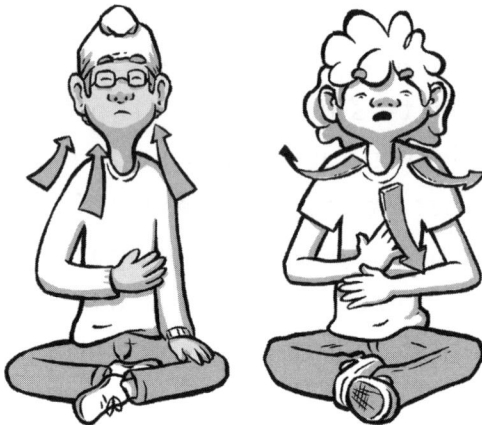

Find a quiet place. You may choose to stand, sit or lie down for this activity. Some people like to use a sound such as a bell or chime at the beginning and end of the exercise. This can help you focus.

Rest both your hands on your belly. You may want to close your eyes. Begin by concentrating on your breath. Just notice how natural breathing is. Become aware of your hands moving each time you breathe in and out. Notice as the air fills your lungs Just breathe in and out... Notice as the air moves naturally through your body. Let each breath sink down deep into your belly. Notice as the air moves through your nose and out through your mouth. Perhaps the air is warm or cold. You may hear the sound of your breath as you inhale and you can pay attention to the rise and fall of your belly. There may be other sounds around you or perhaps your thoughts wander and as you begin to think about other things. That's OK, just bring your attention back to breathing. Notice how it feels to focus all your attention on your breath. In...and...out...

Continue the exercise for one or two minutes before completing the table below. There are no right or wrong answers.

How did the exercise make you feel?	
Which physical sensations did you notice in your body?	
Were you able to stay focused on your breathing or did you have a 'monkey mind'? If you did have a 'monkey mind', what things popped into your mind?	

Mindful chocolate eating

Some people eat food too quickly. Sometimes we even forget what we've eaten. Frequently our minds wander off and we do not really notice the process of eating at all, especially if we are doing another activity at the same time such as watching TV or playing on our phone.

In this exercise, we are going to experiment by eating something differently. Perhaps in a way we have never eaten before. While completing this exercise, focus all of your attention on the chocolate. Imagine you are doing this activity as though it is the first time you have ever seen or eaten chocolate before. Approach the exercise with an open mind and a gentle curiosity.

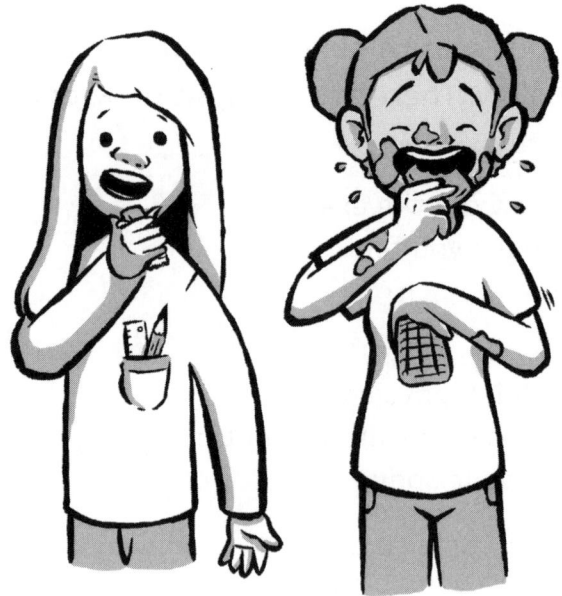

Pick up your chocolate but don't eat it yet. Place it in the palm of your hand and notice its colour and shape. Feel the weight of it in your hand. Pretend you have never seen or eaten chocolate before. Examine the chocolate closely. Touch the chocolate and notice the texture. How does it feel in your fingers? Examine the chocolate, noticing its colour. Look at the different sides of the chocolate and notice how the light reflects on it, or any shadows. If your mind starts to wander and think about other things, that's OK. Notice the thoughts and bring your attention back to the chocolate. You may hear other people or other noises in the room. Notice the sounds and bring your attention back to the chocolate. Raise the chocolate to your nose and smell the chocolate. Slowly breathe in several times and focus on the different smells. Does smelling the chocolate trigger anything else in your body? Is your mouth watering? Are you having any thoughts such as 'What's taking so long?' or 'Hurry up and let me eat the chocolate!'? If so, notice them and bring your attention back to smelling the chocolate. Now slowly take a small bite of the chocolate, but do not chew it or swallow it. Notice the feeling and taste of the chocolate in your mouth. How does it feel as it melts? Notice the taste and sensations of the chocolate on your tongue. Move the chocolate around in your mouth. Notice the moment where you feel like you want to swallow. Slowly swallow the chocolate, focusing on the sensations. Notice any lingering tastes or sensations.

How was this different from your normal way of eating chocolate? What did you notice during the exercise?	
Do you have any ideas about how these principles might apply to eating or other areas of your life?	

Gratitude

Gratitude is part of mindfulness and becoming more aware of yourself and others. It is important to show appreciation and be thankful for all the things we have got rather than focus on what we have not.

It can be useful to shift focus from what you don't have to all the wonderful things you do have. In the box below list or draw some things you are grateful for in your own life. This could include your friends and family, beautiful things in the world around you, or your favourite activities or things to do.

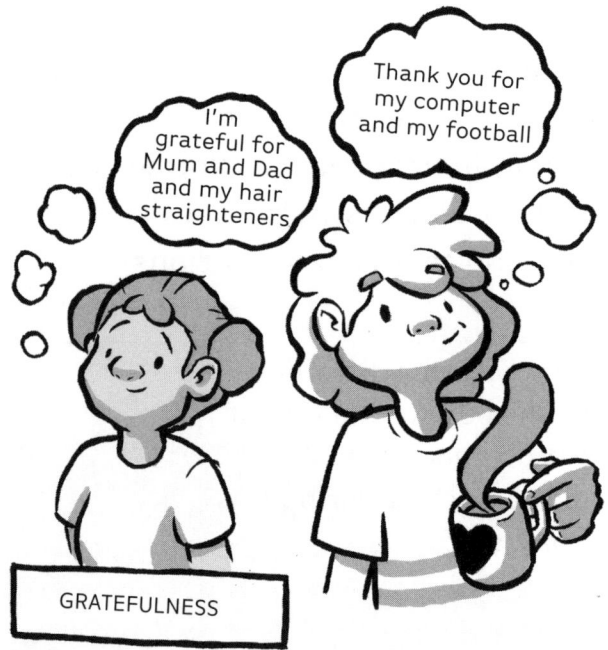

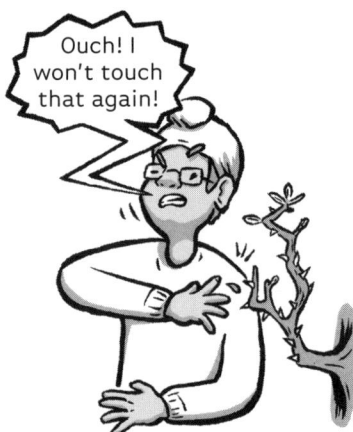

It is also important to be grateful for our thoughts and feelings. Yes, even the ones we do not like or that make us feel uncomfortable, such as anger or fear. The truth is that all our feelings are linked with our survival. All emotions have a positive intention and help us in some way. Our feelings keep us safe, either from a physical threat – for example, something hurting your body – or from psychological threat such as being laughed at or left out of a friendship group.

Imagine what would happen if you could not experience your feelings. For example, imagine if you were not able to experience the emotion of fear. You would not know to keep away from danger. You might even try and make friends with a crocodile. Alternatively, if you could not feel anger, people might take advantage of you or break your things. People are much more prepared to help you if you are thankful for their efforts, and the same thing is true of your own body and feelings.

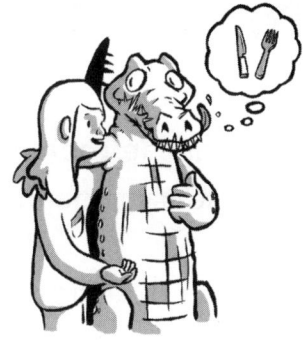

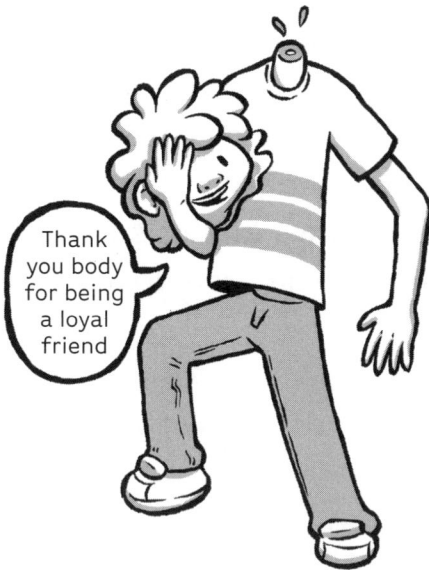

Jack suggests that it is better to be mindful than to lose your head! Our bodies are like a loyal friend working hard to keep us healthy and in balance. Even subconsciously our bodies remind us when we are hungry or thirsty; our body even keeps our hearts beating while we are asleep.

In Session 4 we learned that our body sends alarm signals if it thinks we are in danger.

It also brings feelings of joy and happiness when things go well. Can you think of any other ways your body works for you like a faithful friend to protect and keep you safe?

It is important to be kind to yourself and thank your body for all its hard efforts.

Mindfulness of thoughts and feelings

Explore the roots of your scary thoughts. Bad beliefs should not bear fruit. Stop scary thoughts branching out, let your thoughts be free.

This can be tricky. Some children have very scary or frightening thoughts. They imagine that the worst is going to happen. *Some children even imagine that their thoughts or feelings are powerful or magical.* For example, 'If I think something bad about my family it will come true', or 'If I feel bad it means I am bad'. However, this is not true. The fact is that *thoughts are just thoughts.* There are no good or bad thoughts. Everyone has upsetting thoughts and feelings sometimes. But, just because you have bad or angry feelings, it does not mean you are a bad person. Even your parents, teachers and friends have scary or uncomfortable thoughts and feelings sometimes and this is quite normal. However, it is not what you think or feel but what you do and the actions you take that counts.

Circle or put a tick by the individuals below who are most likely to get into trouble:

Jack thinks his sister is mean. He wishes he could shout at her and push her over.	
Lauren thinks her brother is mean, so she pushes him over.	
Amir blames Katie when he is caught throwing darts at his parents.	
Katie imagines herself stealing her friend's birthday present because it is really cool.	
Amir's dog is hungry so it eats the cat's food, and boy does it taste good.	
Lauren's friend feels angry with her mother. She thinks about being rude to her.	

Mindfulness can be helpful in coping with both our thoughts and feelings. As discussed in Session 10, when we do not like our thoughts and feelings, we avoid them or try and think about something else. This puts pressure on us and we can end up in a battle with ourselves. The more we push our thoughts and feelings away, the more we notice them. You can make cool connections by learning to accept your feelings, which helps you make better choices and feel more comfortable in your body and mind. There are lots of mindful ways to notice your thoughts and feelings (without judgement) and to just let them go. Try the following mindful exercises with your thoughts. This will take practice.

Imagine your thoughts passing through the sky on a banner attached to an aeroplane. Just notice as they slowly move into the distance. Perhaps you could also blow your feelings into an imaginary balloon and watch as your thoughts simply float off into the distance.

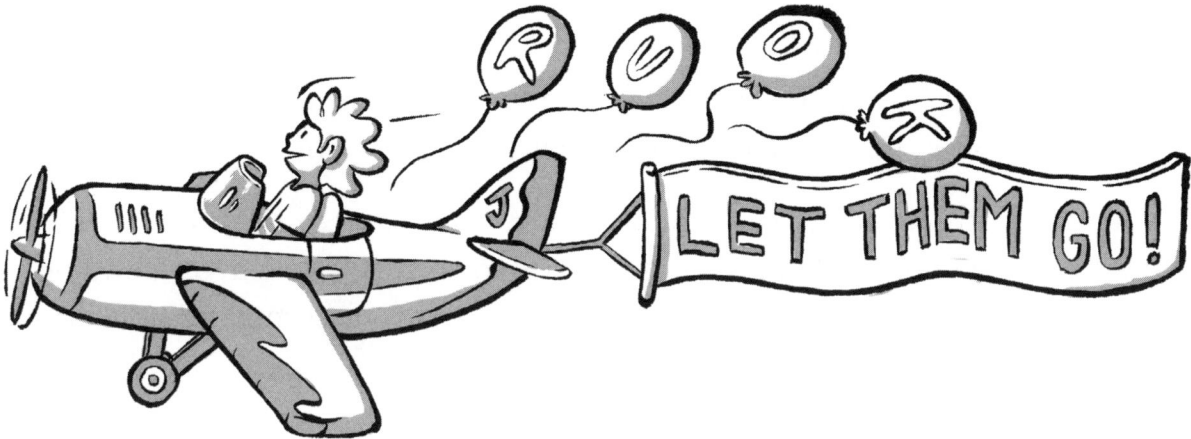

Leaves on a stream visualisation

1. Sit in a comfortable position and either close your eyes or rest them gently on a fixed spot in the room.

2. Visualise yourself sitting beside a gently flowing stream with leaves floating along the surface of the water. *Pause 10 seconds.*

3. For the next few minutes, take each thought that enters your mind and place it on a leaf. Let it float away. Do this with each thought – pleasurable, painful or neutral. Even if you have joyous or enthusiastic thoughts, place them on a leaf and let them float away.

4. If your thoughts momentarily stop, continue to watch the stream. Sooner or later, your thoughts will start up again. *Pause 20 seconds.*

5. Allow the stream to flow at its own pace. Don't try to speed it up and rush your thoughts along. You're not trying to rush the leaves along or 'get rid' of your thoughts. You are allowing them to come and go at their own pace.

6. If your mind says 'This is dumb', 'I'm bored' or 'I'm not doing this right', place those thoughts on leaves, too, and let them float away. *Pause 20 seconds.*

7. If a leaf gets stuck, allow it to hang around until it's ready to float by. If the thought comes up again, watch it float by the second time. *Pause 20 seconds.*

8. If a difficult or painful feeling arises, simply acknowledge it. Say to yourself, 'I notice myself having a feeling of boredom/impatience/frustration.' Place those thoughts on leaves and allow them to float along.

9. From time to time, your thoughts may hook you and distract you from being fully present in this exercise. This is *normal*. As soon as you realise that you have become side-tracked, gently bring your attention back to the visualisation exercise.

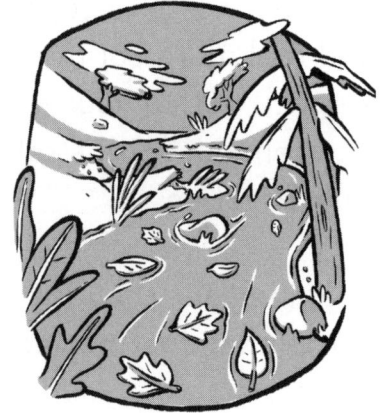

Light stream visualisation

Mindfulness can also be used to help with feelings. The following involves an experiment to test out what happens when we move closer and accept our feelings rather than avoiding or pushing them away.

Write or draw about a recent time when you felt upset. Perhaps you were sad, worried or angry.

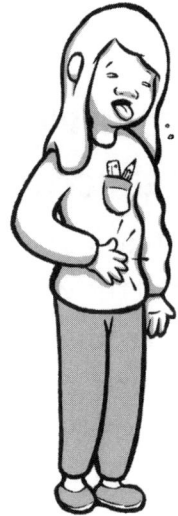

Put your hand on the place you feel the feeling most strongly in your body and answer the following questions. If you are not sure, just make it up. There are no right or wrong answers.

If the feeling had a shape, what would it be?	
If it had a size, how big would it be?	
If it had a colour, what colour would it be?	
Would it be hot or cold?	
Would it be hard, soft, rough or smooth?	
If it had a sound, would it be high or low pitched?	

Now imagine a healing light coming down from above and moving in through the top of your head, and that this healing light is directing itself at the shape in your body. Give this wonderful healing light your favourite colour and notice if it feels warm or cold in your body. Notice as the light fills up your body, moving into every part of the shape and spreading its healing powers. Write in the box below any changes you noticed about the shape and your feelings.

Mindfulness overview

Four elements exercises for stress reduction (earth, air, water, fire)

Stress can build up during the day. The following techniques can help you cope better with stress and help you stay calm and be cool. These ideas were first introduced by an American psychologist called Elan Shapiro in 2012.[1] He has found that if people practise the four elements they are more in control of their emotions and seem to live more balanced lives. Although these exercises seem quite simple, they can be difficult to master and you will need plenty of time to practise.

Earth

GROUNDING, SAFETY in the PRESENT. Take a minute or two to 'land'...to be in the here and now. Place both feet on the ground, feel the chair supporting you. Look around and notice three new things. What do you see? What do you hear?

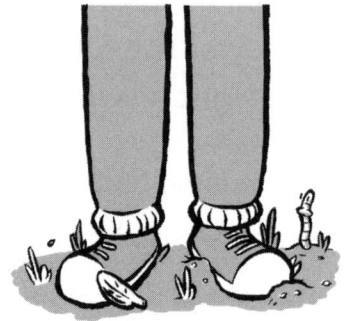

Air

BREATHING for CENTRING your body. Practise the mindful breathing exercise earlier in this session. Remember to breathe in through your nose and out through your mouth. Some people find blowing gently on the nose as you breathe out can be really cool and calming.

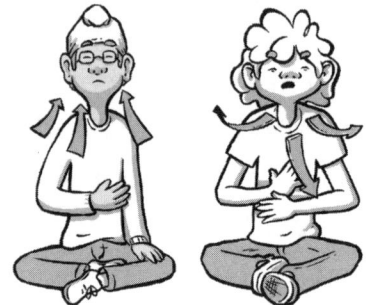

---

1   This exercise has been adapted from Shapiro, E. (2012) '4 Elements Exercise.' *Journal of EMDR Practice and Research*, 1, 2,113–115.

Water

RELAXATION RESPONSE. Do you have saliva in your mouth? When you are anxious or stressed, your mouth often dries out as part of the stress response. Making saliva in your mouth is also a way of calming your mind and body. Drinking water is thought to be helpful too, and stops you becoming dehydrated.

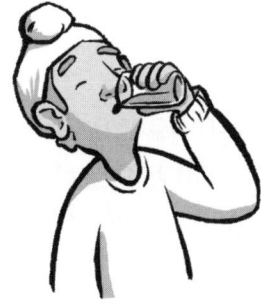

Fire or light

Draw a safe calm place like a tropical beach. LIGHT up the path of your IMAGINATION. Bring up an image of your safe place (or some other resource such as a memory when you felt good about yourself) – what do you feel and where do you feel it in your body?

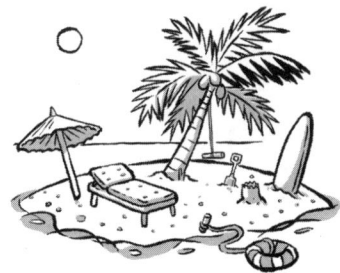

Some children like to make a bracelet or neckless with different colours or beads to remind them of the different elements above.

Home activity 12: Mindfulness experiment

Everything we do can be done mindfully. This week experiment while doing some other day-to-day tasks mindfully such as brushing your teeth, running a race or even 'tidying your bedroom'. Perhaps that's just going too far! The key to becoming a master of mindfulness is to practise, practise, practise. *Mindfully of course!*

In the table below, list some things you did mindfully this week. What did you notice...?

Mindful activity	What did you notice?

SESSION 13: MORE COOL CONNECTIONS

Aims and objectives

- Learn new cool ways of coping.

- Enhance the skills the group has already learned.

Materials

Pens or pencils.

Agenda and tips for running the session

All of the exercises in this session are useful. However, after reading through 'More of what matters', you will find that most of the skills and information in this part of the programme have been shared in some way previously in the book. Consequently, it is at the facilitator's discretion which parts to leave out if a shorter session is required. While 'Five ways to personal well-being' is a useful exercise, group members may find the 'Magic card challenge' more engaging and fun. Many children also value the information on magical thinking, but this was partly covered in Session 12.

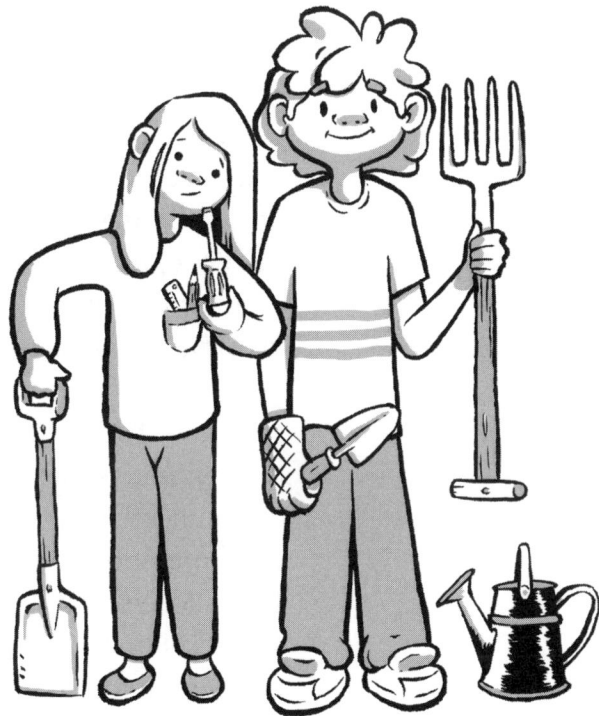

Short session

EXERCISE	COMMENT
Welcome children	Share agenda for Session 13 with the group.
Review Home activity 12	The group members briefly show how they completed homework tasks and share this with the rest of the group. Note the different activities chosen. How easy or difficult were the activities to complete? What did the children learn?
More of what matters	Keeping active and doing pleasurable activities is important to both increase and maintain well-being. Unfortunately, when people struggle with their emotions or become low in mood, they tend to stop doing things they used to enjoy and often avoid social interaction. This exercise is not just about encouraging individuals to do more, but to increase activities that matter to them, including things they enjoy. Sometimes individuals find it difficult to name any activities they enjoy. It may be necessary to list things they enjoyed in the past or to speak with their friends and family to help with this. It may be useful to ask, 'If you didn't have any current difficulties, how would you spend your time, or what would you enjoy doing on your own, or with friends or family?' This exercise also involves making some concrete plans about when/how the individual will complete the activity. Many individuals will need their parents to help with this task. Parents are usually more than happy to help.
Making good use of your time	Encourage individuals to read through the text. Some children will need their parents to help out with this task, which can be completed as the home activity.
Five ways to personal well-being	This exercise speaks for itself. Some children may benefit from taking a copy of this page home with them to remember the CLEAN acronym.

Magical thinking
A magical thinking style is very common with people experiencing anxiety. It may be useful to list examples of this thinking style or share further examples through discussion. The first step to help children is to help them become aware of when they are using a magical thinking style.

Magic card challenge
The purpose of this exercise is to help children see in a fun way that it is not possible to predict the future. Some children believe their thoughts are powerful and they can make things happen just by thinking about them. This experiment helps test this theory and can open up further discussion.

Window breathing
There are numerous breathing exercises teaching children to relax. This idea is simple and easy to use.

Moving feelings
This is similar to the 'Light stream visualisation' in Session 12 in which it is described how children tend to avoid their feelings. Psychologists have found that by validating and accepting/acknowledging our feelings we have a greater sense of control and well-being. Some children may find this difficult, while to others it will make perfect sense. If children struggle, just help them to notice and accept that this is okay and move on in the book.

Thumbs up!
Many people find it helpful to externalise their worries. This often helps children separate their thoughts and feelings. Obviously, any part of the body or even a toy can be used rather than the children's thumbs.

Home activity 13: Magical thinking
Individuals are encouraged to notice people's magical thinking style. This can also increase self-awareness if they include themselves. An alternative to this home activity could be practising one of the other activities in this session and feeding back in the next session. Some facilitators might like to give children the choice of a home activity following this session.

Long session

More time can be spent discussing each exercise with the group. It may also be fun for the children to find a partner and role play some of the activities to share with the group. The group could spend time drawing or discussing things that are important to them, or find pictures from magazines. Group members could also practise some of the techniques such as 'Window breathing' as a group together. As suggested in Session 12, there are a number of short YouTube videos which can be viewed linked with the ideas in this session. Facilitators can search topics such as magical thinking, or well-being cartoons for kids, for additional ideas.

Notes

The exercises in this session are aimed at providing additional tools to help increase well-being and resilience. The exercises build on many of those already covered in the programme. As well as drawing on literature about CBT, some of these exercises also draw from other therapeutic approaches such as behavioural activation (BA), and ideas adapted from EMDR and NLP therapies.

More of what matters

Scientists have noticed that when people feel down or upset they do less of the things they used to enjoy. They describe life as 'boring' and they find it more difficult to have fun. Consequently, people do less and spend more time alone and away from other people. Some individuals find they just can't be bothered to do anything and spend lots of time thinking about negative things. Life becomes like wearing the gloomy cap discussed in Session 7. The problem is, the more we avoid people and the less we do, the fewer opportunities there are for changing the way we feel. Therefore, over time we remain stuck in a negative cycle. See the chart below.

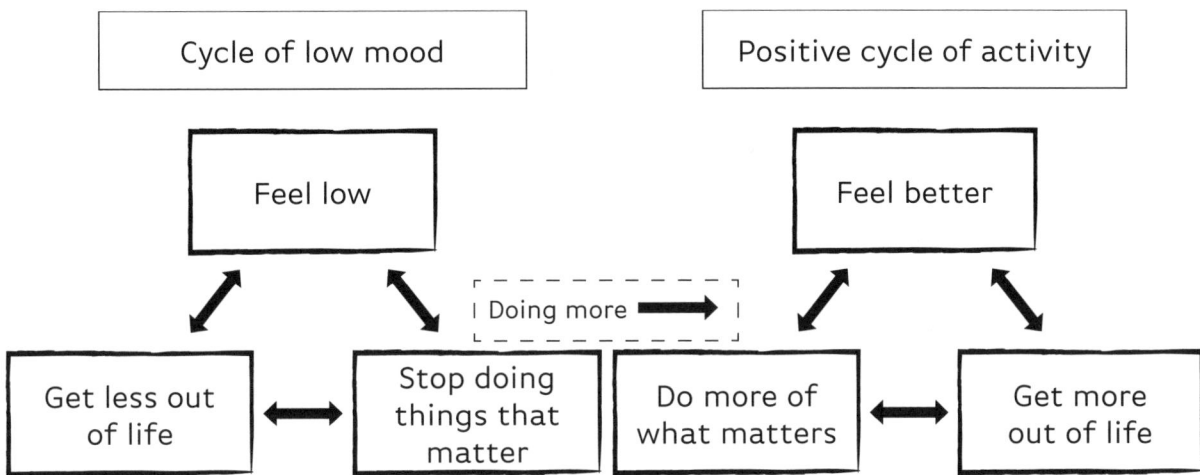

Cycle of low mood	Positive cycle of activity

Feel low

Doing more ➡

Feel better

Get less out of life ⬌ Stop doing things that matter

Do more of what matters ⬌ Get more out of life

The truth is, the more we do of what matters to us the better we feel. This is not the same as 'just doing more activities'. This is about finding the things that matter or are important to you and spending more time doing them. Doctors have noted that doing more of what people enjoy actually changes people's brains, making them more healthy, as well as increasing feelings of well-being and happiness.

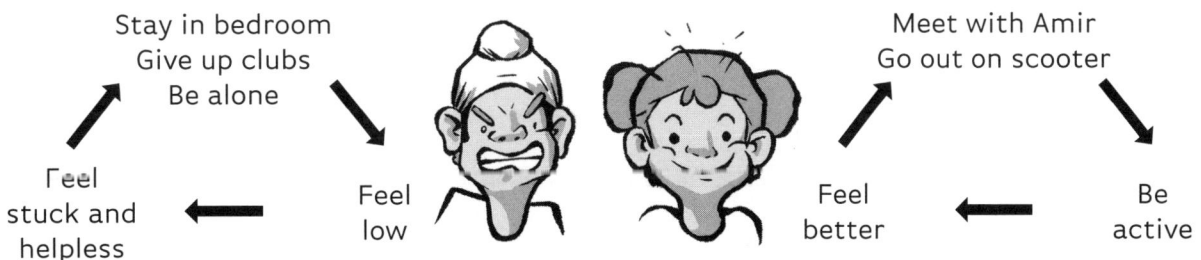

Stay in bedroom
Give up clubs
Be alone

Meet with Amir
Go out on scooter

Feel stuck and helpless

Feel low

Feel better

Be active

In the following box, you are encouraged to list things which matter or are important to you (your values).

Circle two things from your list. Make a plan about how you can do more of these things over the next two weeks. Be clear and specific, as learned in Session 9. It is better to choose things that can be achieved yourself rather than activities that require help or money from a grown-up. Simple activities are best. See Lauren and Amir's plans below:

Lauren plans to invite Katie to play on Saturday and will colour in her book every day after school.

Amir has agreed to play football at break times in school and walk his dog every morning.

Now complete your own plans in the box below.

What are your plans? When/how will you make them happen?

Making good use of your time

Our brain gets a boost when we achieve things during the day. Achievement increases the feel-good factor in our brains. It is therefore very helpful to plan goals every day to help us feel better about ourselves and the world around us. Just increasing our activity and exercise levels can make us feel better about ourselves and life in general. Some people find it useful to plan their week in advance. This can really help lift your mood. By using a diary to plan your week in advance, you may be able to do more of the things that matter to you as well as doing the 'boring stuff' you need to do. Research has found that planning ahead can really help lift your mood. You could also make a weekly plan by using the 'Activity and feelings record' from Session 3.

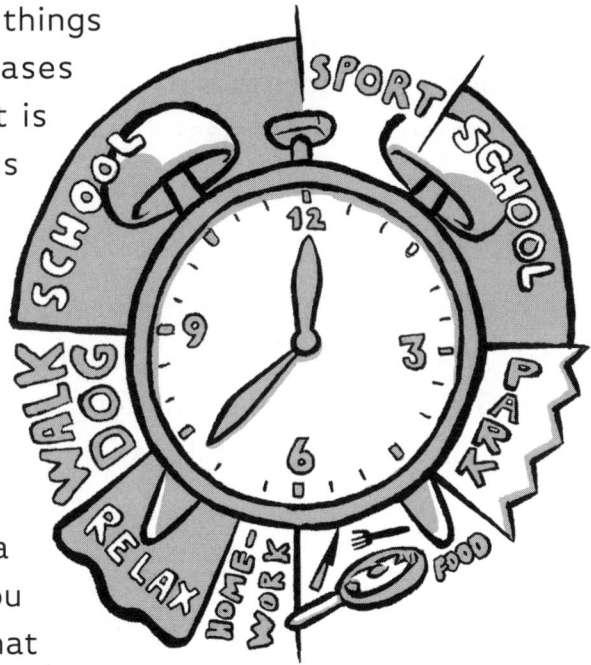

A question of balance

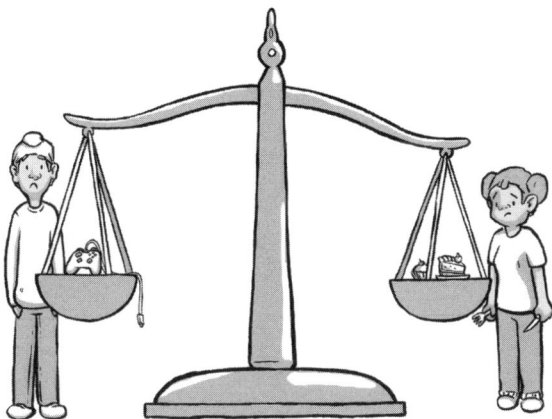

Having a balance in life is important. For example, sweets and cakes are very important to Katie, but if she eats too many this may not be good for her. Amir loves his computer, but if he spends all day in his bedroom he won't have the chance to go out with his friends.

Interacting with other people

As well as activities, mixing with other people is also important. When people feel low or worried they tend to hide away and keep themselves to themselves. The problem is that the more we avoid things and hide away from others, the more lonely we become and we can become increasingly stuck – like a never-ending cycle of gloominess.

Experiment

Try interacting with three different people and notice how they respond and how this makes you feel. You could try saying hello or even just giving them a smile. Giving others a compliment is another way to make yourself and others feel good. There is a popular saying, 'Smile and the world smiles with you'.

Five ways to personal well-being – CLEAN

Connect

Make time to be with your family and friends. Make contact with others at home, school and in your local neighbourhood.

Learn

Try something new. Set yourself a challenge. Take up a new hobby, join a club, learn to play an instrument or learn a new language or skill. Be creative!

Exercise

Be active. Get some physical exercise. Get outside. Walk, run, cycle, swim, play, work out, garden or dance.

Acts of kindness

Give. Do something nice for your parents, teacher, a friend or even your pets. Say thank you or just smile at others. Do something to help someone else either at home, school or in your community, providing you have your parents' permission.

Notice

Be curious. Become aware and take notice of your environment. Catch sight of things that are beautiful in the world and savour each moment.

Magical thinking

Everyone has thoughts and feelings linked with the past, present and future. Some of these thoughts are very useful because they can motivate us and make us feel good. As we have learned in this book, our thoughts affect the way that we feel. But, our thoughts are not always true. There are two unhelpful styles which can cause some people to feel very stuck and confused. These thinking styles include mind reading and fortune telling:

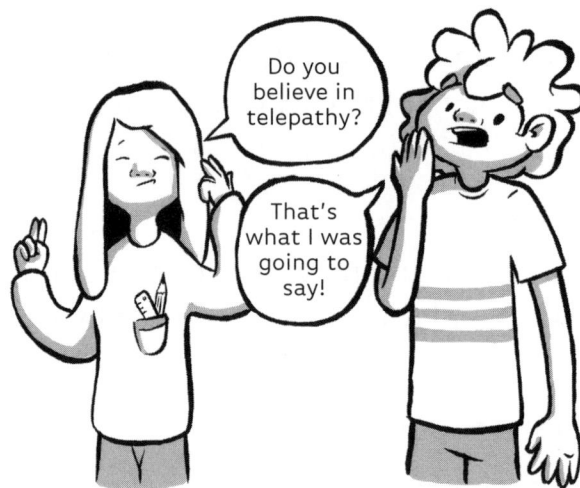

Mind reading: Mind reading is when you think that you know what everyone else is thinking. For example: 'Everyone hates Katie because she's so brainy', or 'All the boys think Amir is cool for being rude to the teachers'.

Fortune telling: Fortune telling is when you act as though you already know what will happen in the future. For example: 'Jack missed a penalty kick in the last match, so he will definitely miss again if he takes another penalty', or 'Mum will kill me if I tell her how I feel'. While it is possible that the above statements are true, it is also possible that they may not be. Unless we are magical or can time travel, most people can't see into the future.

Don't believe everything you think!

Just because you think something, it does not mean that it is going to happen or that your thoughts are true. Unless you have magical powers, your thoughts and feelings cannot cause bad things to happen. Thoughts are just thoughts. Some people think they're especially magical, believing that their thoughts are powerful and they can make things happen just by thinking about them. For example, it is quite common for people to have thoughts such as: 'If I think bad thoughts about someone then something bad will happen', or 'If I think I am going to win the lottery I will have a better chance of winning'.

Often children have unhelpful magical-type thoughts about themselves too, such as 'I am weird, odd, ugly or different. I think this, therefore it must be true.' We often believe these thoughts without any real evidence to back them up. See if you can think of an example of magical-type thinking and write or draw it in the box below:

Although it's quite normal for people to have some magical thoughts from time to time, just thinking about them can't make them happen. To test out this theory, take part in the 'Magic card challenge' with the rest of the group. You could also try this experiment with a partner, friend or family member.

Magic card challenge

This is an experiment to test the magical powers of your thinking. Can you tell if a card is *black* or *red* just by thinking about it? To take the test you will need a partner and a pack of ordinary playing cards for this experiment (remove the jokers from the pack before you start).

- Deal 21 cards on the table without looking at them.

- Partner one picks up 21 cards from the table to test the magical thinking powers of their friend.

- Partner two must guess the colour of the cards one by one by saying 'black' or 'red'.

- If partner two guesses correctly, the cards are placed in one pile. If they get the colour wrong, the card is placed in a separate pile. Do not let your partner know which pile is which until the experiment is complete.

- Swap roles and let partner one test the power of his/her thoughts with the cards.

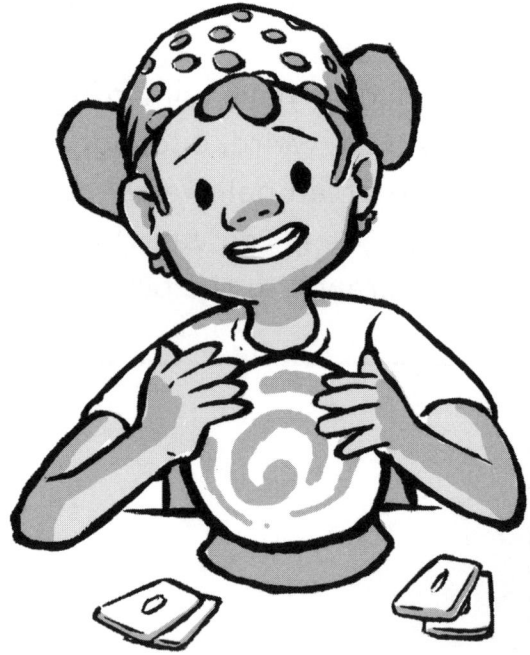

If you don't get at least 19 correct every time, I think that we can safely say that your thoughts are not powerful and you can't make things happen just by thinking about them!

Window breathing

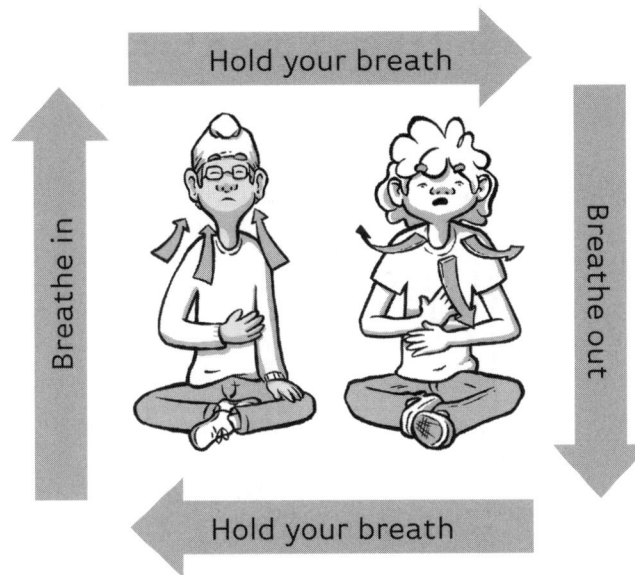

In Session 4, you learned about body signals and the effect breathing has on our bodies. The window breathing technique is another helpful way of getting your breathing into a more rhythmical pattern and helping you feel more relaxed and calm.

- Sit in a comfortable position, then start by focusing on a rectangular object. Windows are a good example, but it could be any rectangle such as your TV, computer or even a table or desk in your classroom at school.

- Start by looking along the short edge, breathing in (inhaling) through your nose as you do so.

- When you reach the longest length, breathe out, exhaling from your mouth as your eyes follow the line down.

- Do this along the other sides, remembering to breathe in on the short sides and breathe out on the longer ones.

- Repeat until your breathing returns to normal and you feel calm and relaxed.

The idea in the picture below can also be helpful when thinking about changing your breathing and the effect this has on your body.

When I take a deep breath

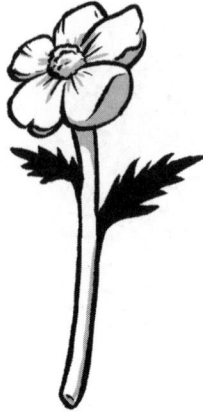

I smell a
flower

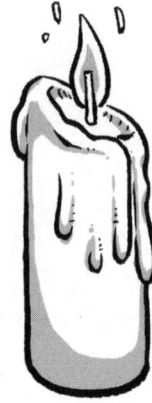

Then blow out
a candle

Moving feelings

In Session 3, we learned about the importance of feeling our emotions, but we tend to avoid feelings when they are uncomfortable. The trouble is that the more we avoid the way we feel, the more stuck we can become. The following exercise externalises feelings that are uncom-fortable and can help you feel more in control of your emotions. Think of a time when you had a strong uncomfortable emotion, such as when you experienced fear, sadness, jealousy or anger. In the accompanying picture, notice where Katie and Amir have located their uncomfortable feelings and where they feel the emotion in their bodies. Katie's is a blobby shape, which she describes as red. Amir has a more jagged spotted shape, which he feels in his stomach.

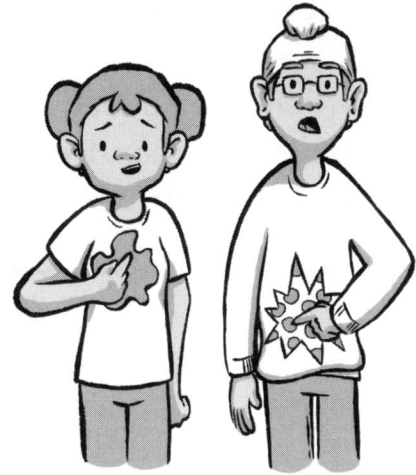

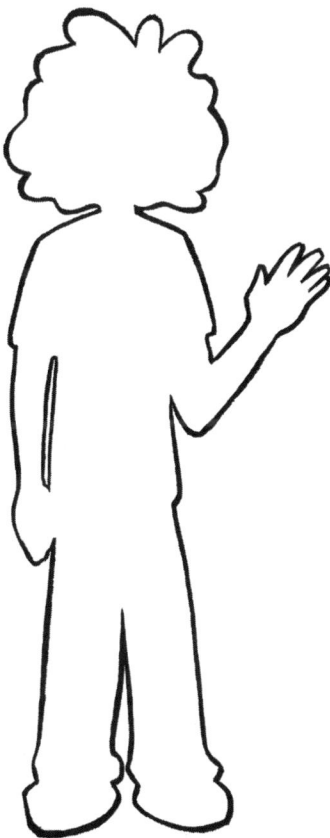

Give your feeling a shape and colour/draw it on the person to the left. Sometimes simply noticing your thoughts and feelings can make you feel different and help bring about change. Notice the feeling for a moment, including its shape and colour. Just repeat what you experience to yourself: 'I am aware that I am feeling sad, scared, lonely and so on.' Write or draw on the person any changes you may experience when you notice your feelings. Experiment by changing the colour and shape. Perhaps move the shape you have drawn to a different part of your body. Just notice if changing the colour or moving the location of your upset feeling makes any difference to the way you think or feel.

Some people describe their feelings as moving inside them, while others report their uncomfortable feelings are motionless and a bit like a 'blob'.

For people whose feelings are still, it can be useful to imagine giving their feeling some movement. Perhaps making it smaller, spinning it around or moving it away from your heart or tummy and placing it in your little finger or big toe.

If your emotion already has movement, it can be useful to slow it down or change its direction. Experiment with your feelings and note any observations or changes in the box below.

Thumbs up!

Most people are lost in their own secret world of thoughts. Thoughts about the world, what they're doing at work or school, and most of all about themselves. The truth is that most people spend many hours each day pondering over various issues, often without being fully aware of the content of their thoughts. As we have already learned, if we want to change the way we feel, we first need to become aware of our thoughts.

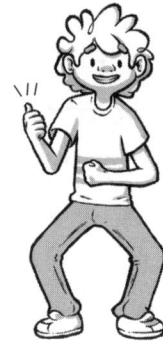

In the following exercise, you make cool connections by doing something different. Practising this exercise will help distance you from your thoughts and help you feel calmer and more in control. Because this exercise is a bit silly, it can also be helpful because it is not possible to laugh and feel upset at the same time.

Imagine moving your negative self-talk out of your head, down your arm to the end of your thumb. Put your thumb up and imagine saying some of the mean things you say to yourself from your thumb. This may seem a bit strange at first. Go ahead and change the sound of the mean or negative things you say to yourself into something ridiculous, such as a cartoon character. Perhaps make it squeaky! See what happens when you say mean things to yourself in a silly voice from the end of your thumb.

You may begin to notice that although the words you are saying are the same, they just don't feel so bad. You may even find yourself chuckling to yourself. But, don't laugh too loud or people might notice, especially if you're seen talking to your thumb in public! The more you do the exercise, the more it will become automatic. Another variation of the above could be to imagine your phone is talking to you in a silly voice. Imagine Siri has malfunctioned and turned into Donald Duck while you are taking a selfie.

Home activity 13: Catch magical thinking

In the table below, see if you can catch occasions when people are using a magical thinking style. Write the name of the person in the column on the left and what they have said in the column on the right. For example, 'My friend Ahmed' and 'You will definitely get an A in your spelling test'. You can also include your own thoughts – it's your choice.

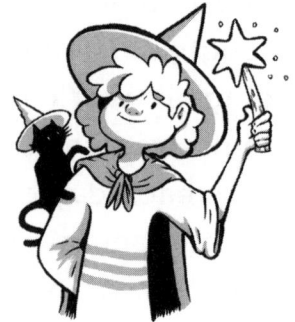

Person's name	Magical thinking statement

SESSION 14: EVALUATION

Aims and objectives

- Evaluate the programme.

- Find out what we have learned.

- See if the group has helped with your feelings.

- Find some ideas on how to improve the group for other children in the future.

- Congratulate each other on completing the programme and receive a certificate.

Materials

Chairs, pencils.

Agenda and tips for running the session

Exercises in bold in the left-hand column should be included in both long and short sessions. Many fun activities and games are included as optional. Despite sometimes being short of time it is important not to cut all the 'fun' out of the programme or you will lose the children's enthusiasm.

Short session

EXERCISE	COMMENT
Feedback	Welcome the children and share agenda for session with the group. Obtain brief feedback from the children's week.
Review Home activity 13	Children can share and discuss their home activities. Children are encouraged to show or perform their home activity in front of the group.
Game	Children are invited to choose one or two of the games played in sessions earlier in the programme.
Re-rate yourself	Children are encouraged to re-rate themselves. Compare the ratings with the same exercise in Session 1. It is useful to discuss with the children what they make of any changes that have taken place. What have they learned/experienced to contribute to the change in the rating scores?
Cool connections evaluation	Children complete the 'Cool connections evaluation'. The first seven questions reflect the basic aims and objectives of the programme. Children are encouraged to add any further comments if they wish.

Long session

You may wish to include a mini-party as a celebration for completing the programme. This could include cakes, drinks and so on. You may wish to make your own certificates and present them to the children.

Notes

In some cases when the children re-rate themselves, the level of fear or upset may appear to have got worse since the beginning of the programme. This does not matter. It is only a measure. It is possible that a child's personal/ environmental circumstances may have changed to influence their feelings. For example, during the programme they may have experienced a significant loss or trauma. Some children have also reported that as the programme progressed they learned more about their feelings and were better able to give an accurate measure of their feelings by the end of the programme. This indicates that the measures recorded at the beginning of the programme were inaccurate.

Re-rate yourself

Mark a cross on the number you currently feel most represents your life and how you are coping both in and out of school.

| 1 | 2 | 3 | 4 | 5 | 6 | 7 | 8 | 9 | 10 |

VERY UPSET   **HAPPY**

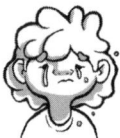

List the three things below which you felt most upset about in your life at the beginning of the programme. (You may need to refer back to the rating in Session 1.) Put a cross on the number which best represents how you feel now.

Example: I have not got many friends

| 1 | ✗2 | 3 | 4 | 5 | 6 | 7 | 8 | 9 | 10 |

VERY UPSET   **HAPPY**

1: . . . .

| 1 | 2 | 3 | 4 | 5 | 6 | 7 | 8 | 9 | 10 |

VERY UPSET   **HAPPY**

2: . . . .

| 1 | 2 | 3 | 4 | 5 | 6 | 7 | 8 | 9 | 10 |

VERY UPSET   **HAPPY**

3: . . . .

| 1 | 2 | 3 | 4 | 5 | 6 | 7 | 8 | 9 | 10 |

VERY UPSET   **HAPPY**

Cool connections evaluation

For each of the following questions please put a tick in the boxes below.

Have you had fun in the group?

Not at all	A little bit	A lot	Loads

Has being in the group helped you get on better with other children?

Not at all	A little bit	A lot	Very much

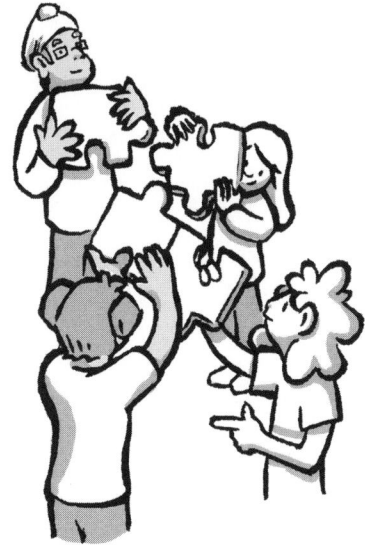

Has being in the group helped you feel more confident?

Not at all	A little bit	A lot	Very much

Has being in the group given you new experiences?

Not at all	A little bit	A lot	Loads

Do you think that the group has helped you feel better about yourself?

Not at all	A little bit	A lot	Very much

Has being in the group helped you with your worries?

Not at all	A little bit	A lot	Very much

What would you tell other children about the group?

Load of rubbish	It was OK	Very good	Super cool and brilliant

Further comments about the group: